OCCUPATIONAL
CANCER

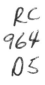

THE NATURE OF
OCCUPATIONAL
CANCER

A CRITICAL REVIEW OF
PRESENT PROBLEMS

By

BERTRAM D. DINMAN, M.D., Sc. D.

Director
Institute of Environmental and Industrial Health
The University of Michigan
School of Public Health
Ann Arbor, Michigan

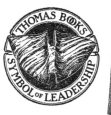

CHARLES C THOMAS • PUBLISHER
Springfield • Illinois • U.S.A.

Published and Distributed Throughout the World by

CHARLES C THOMAS • PUBLISHER
Bannerstone House
301-327 East Lawrence Avenue, Springfield, Illinois, U.S.A.

© *1974 by* CHARLES C THOMAS • PUBLISHER
ISBN 0-398-02907-5
Library of Congress Catalog Card Number 73-7804

*With THOMAS BOOKS careful attention is given to all details of
manufacturing and design. It is the Publisher's desire to present books that
are satisfactory as to their physical qualities and artistic possibilities and
appropriate for their particular use. THOMAS BOOKS will be true to those
laws of quality that assure a good name and good will.*

Library of Congress Cataloging in Publication Data
Dinman, Bertram D
    The nature of occupational cancer.

    1. Occupational diseases. 2. Cancer. 3. Carcinogens. I. Title. [DNLM: 1.
Neoplasms. 2: Occupational diseases: QZ 200 D585o 1973] RC964.D5 616.9'94'071
73-7804 ISBN 0-398-02907-5

Printed in the United States of America
HH-11

ACKNOWLEDGMENT

I WISH TO EXPRESS MY appreciation to Dr. Luigi Parmeggiani, former Chief, Safety and Health Branch, ILO, for his kind permission to utilize the material compiled in preparation of a monograph on Occupational Cancer for the International Labor Office, to access to files of his Organization regarding Occupational Cancer and to his staff for their advice, consultation and *informal* translations.

CONTENTS

OCCUPATIONAL CANCER

Chapter I

THE NATURE OF OCCUPATIONAL CANCER

GENERAL BIOLOGIC CONSIDERATIONS

C ANCER OCCURS UNIVERSALLY in time and place, since the neoplastic process is intimately associated with aberrations in fundamental processes regulating cellular replication, growth and organization. Because such activities are basic to life itself, wherever there is life, there appears to be a risk of cancer developing. Since we barely perceive the outlines of the basic processes governing cellular activity, we likewise barely comprehend the neoplastic process. As regards occupation induced cancer, our grasp of this particular phenomenon suffers the same inadequacies as our understanding of the neoplastic process per se. Nevertheless, sufficient data is presently available which clearly associates neoplasia with environmental agents peculiar to the workplace.

While causality attributable to specific exogenous agents is well established, one cannot disregard the role of intrinsic factors in cancer induction. There appears to be an involvement of the genetic material of the cell with cancerous change. It is not clear whether this bespeaks direct aberration of hereditary material, i.e., a *genetic change,* or an alteration of nongenetic material which affects the hereditary material, i.e., an *epigenetic change.* It is well-established that aberrant chromosomal replications occur constantly, e.g., in 0.3 percent of normally dividing leucocytes (Bloom, et al.) Assuming that few of such cells survive, and given the number of replicative events occurring in a lifetime, it would seem that somatic mutation might be an important determinant of carcinogenic alteration. However, there is little evidence at present that such somatic mutation *per se* is necessary for cancer causation. For example, retinoblastoma, while due to a hereditary mutation of a single gene which is present in *all* cells of the individual, does not cause generalized carcinogenic stimulus. The direct cause of retinoblastoma is in epigenetic events favored by general metabolic activities determined by that mutated gene. In sum, at this time the somatic mutation theory has remained unsubstantiated.

However, other internally mediated events appear to be determinants of malignant transformations, e.g. endogenous modifiers such as oestrogenic substances, interactions with interferon and other immunologically active agents, etc. Less readily perceived are the factors responsible for individual variations in metabolic degradative pathways which may affect the results of the contact with carginogens. To take a dichotomous position, the near-universality of cancer could suggest either the existence of an extremely wide-spread distribution and diversity of environmental carcinogens, or multifarious endogenous potentials for neoplastic alteration common to the life process itself.

In fact, probably both environmental and endogenous factors are both operative. Cancer is world-wide, being among the three leading causes of death in persons over 44 years of age (WHO Statistics Reports). Geographic variations in organ-site involvement (Dunham and Bailar) have suggested possibilities of cancer induction by environmental carcinogens differentially distributed; this *inter alia,* does not eliminate the possibility of genetic pool variations in susceptibility. Temporal and spatial variations in the prevalence of, e.g. bronchiogenic or gastrointestinal cancer, have been discussed at length by Hueper, yet for many of his arguments for unique exogenous causality there are equally adequate contradictory positions taken. For example, the absence of pulmonary adenomata in both control and urethane-treated white-footed field-mice suggests that the "induction of such tumors" is dependent upon the existence of endogenous tendencies for these to arrive (Gross *et al,* 1967). By contrast, Shubik and co-workers have induced tumors of a type never seen in a species of control animals utilized in their study.

However, considerable caution must be exercised before attributing carcinogenesis to genetic pool variations. Such an approach is attractive in attempting to explain the relatively high incidence of primary hepatic cancers among Africans; the fact remains that among American negroes derived from such stock, hepatic neoplasm rates are no different from those of their white neighbors. Clearly, animal experimentation demonstrates the role of genetic determinants on carcinogenesis; attribution of a similar role in humans (used as a convenient explanation in the absence of any others) carries with it the risk of overlooking the existence of a preventable enviromental association.

The foregoing discussions should serve to illuminate the problem of differentiating the occupational cancer from the *naturally occurring,* even at the most simple level (i.e. the assumption of total endogenous causality of tumor induction among workers exposed to carcinogens). In view of these potentials for endogenous causation any superimposition of an enviromental carcinogen must be considered as presenting an additional risk.

Comparisons of Occupational and "Naturally Occurring" Cancers

Examination of other aspects of the biological behaviour of tumors of whatever origin is no more illuminating for the purpose of differentiating occupational from *naturally occurring* tumors. The morphology—gross, cellular, subcellular—of industrial tumors, their metabolic properties—all of these are essentially identical to their non-industrial counterpart. The increasing evidence suggestive of a long-time span of development, e.g. the 10 year average between cervical carcinoma *in situ* (Graham *et al.*) and the appearance of clinical malignancy parallels the notoriously long latent period for most occupational tumors. While admittedly this analogy may not be totally appropriate, observations regarding the period of time between the first malignant cellular alteration and clinical maligancy are necessarily sparse.

Indeed, if one surveys the biology of occupational cancers and compares these with other cancers, one finds few differences except for the commonplace statement that the former tend to be multicentric. This characteristic has long been described for occupational bladder tumors (Washburne), cancers in the lungs of the

Schneeburg miners (Schmorl) and among the skin cancers of mule spinners (Henry and Irvine). While skin cancers of unexposed areas appears consistently unicentric, whether occupational bladder and lung tumors are uniquely multicentric is open to question. Moertel *et al.* have observed that multicentric foci are not uncommon for the *usual* bladder tumor, while similar reports applicable to lung cancers (Cahan *et al.*) exist. Further complicating the question are such considerations as the differentiation of multicentricity from sub-surface extensions or eruptions, as well as other variations in criteria used by various authors for the definition of multicentricity. Among patients with cancers occurring at inaccessible sites, few of these are subject to a long period of observation, e.g. as by routine cystoscopy among dye-intermediate workers. Accordingly, the earliest stage of development of non-occupational tumors are rarely described. Hence, even this frequent statement that occupational cancers are almost uniquely multifocal may be open to question. Once more, the truth probably rests somewhere between the extreme positions, i.e. critical review of the literature suggests that the incidence of multicentric occupational tumor is probably quantitatively greater than among other tumors.

THE ATTRIBUTION OF CANCER TO OCCUPATION

General Limitations Inherent in Presently Available Investigational Techniques

The point of the foregoing discussion of the biology of cancer and its induction is to emphasize our present state of ignorance of the neoplastia process. We cannot comprehend the dynamics of naturally occurring cancer, in addition, we are faced with the "universality of occurrence" of the malignant process. Thus the problem of absolutely attributing occupational risk of cancer to specific jobs is made more difficult, for it seems inevitable that a number of such malignant events will occur regardless of work eposure. Secondly, there is little to differentiate the occupational cancer from other tumors on the basis of biological behaviour. Yet despite these problems of differentiation it is well established that cancers do occur in association with exposure to specific chemical and physical agents encountered in the workplace. While demonstration of this fact has been more readily accomplished as regards some of the more potential carcinogens, it is when dealing with the relatively less potent agents that these problems of differentiation will become even more apparent.

The possible methods of investigations which provide such hints of occupational causation are described below. Suffice to say, the epidemiological approach suffers from a need for systematic accumulation of events which—in the case of occupational cancers induced by weak carcinogens—requires relatively large populations. This follows because a *natural* prevalence of cancers will occur; thus small increments of occurrence are difficult to perceive except among extremely large populations. This also carries the implication that epidemiology more readily provides answers only for relatively potent carcinogenic agents. Another shortcoming—which is augmented by the need for many years of observation of large populations—is that the epidemiological approach provides *post hoc* answers at the cost of human wastage.

Regarding the experimental induction of cancer, this provides numerous problems since the biological phenomena revealed may or may not have parallels in human experience (Cf. summary of Tannenbaum regarding the multiplicity of organ sites of neoplasia in urethane-treated animals). Nevertheless, despite the multitude of questions raised by a wide diversity of methodologies, use of the experimental method has provided us with two immensely useful facts: human cancers can be and are reproduced in animal models, and the existence of a compound's neoplastic induction capacity in animals is a warning which society cannot ignore with impunity.

In summary, the problems of attribution of cancer to occupational exposure suffers from both shortcomings in our experimental approaches (epidemiologic, experimental) and our understanding of the neoplastic process. Accordingly, the ultimate question of occupational attribution in man cannot be totally answered in well controlled laboratory settings; by contrast, while epidemiology should provide answers regarding human cancer experience, given the multitude of poorly discerned variables operating in an uncontrollable setting, this method similarly yields less than perfect answers. It appears that given these imperfect tools, and with a clear understanding of their shortcomings, that both techniques must be jointly and carefully used by scientifically spohisticated researchers and those having responsibility for control of this problem.

Epidemiologic Evaluation of Occupational Exposure

EPIDEMIOLOGIC METHODS AND OCCUPATIONAL CANCER—Reports regarding the induction of occupational cancer essentially take two forms, viz., the epidemiological and the case (or individual) medical report. The discussion which follows assumes some knowledge of epidemiologic principles as outlined in any standard reference text on that subject.

The epidemiological method was first utilized during the last century largely in response to the need to define the effect of biologic pathogens upon human health. Then, this method usually had the advantage of dealing with an apparent one-for-one relationship, i.e. a single agent associated with a discrete, single disease entity. Thus by careful application of epidemiological methods, close *associations* between single environmental agents or vehicles and disease could be demonstrated.

However, as long as the variables in the host-agent interaction were not too numerous, epidemiology served as a powerful tool leading to the isolation of a few such variables and their subsequent laboratory modeling. It gradually became apparent that other variables (e.g. dosage, nutritional status, etc.) could affect the outcome of the host-pathogen encounter. Today, this approach is still highly relevant to occupational health needs. However, recognition of the multitude of variables which affect the man-environment interaction should cause one to consider critically simple theories of causality. Nowhere is this more necessary than in cancer epidemiology.

From such considerations it should be apparent that unless an extremely potent carcinogen is involved, or an unusually large population is at risk, other interacting or concurrent variables tend to obscure the host-agent reaction. Further complicating this interaction is the period of latency which intervenes between exposure and detection of the neoplastic event. Aside from problems of defining what constitutes the line of demarcation between hyperplastic and neoplastic cells, apparent individual variations in response to a carcinogen may cloud the issue. That such variability is not hypothetical is clearly apparent from experimental studies, e.g. all animals exposed to potent carcinogens do not *simultaneously* develop tumors; not *all persons* who smoke for comparable periods subsequently develop lung cancer. Finally, since a multiplicity of materials, known and hypothetical, can act as promotors, a poorly defined universe of environmental agents might be operating, either as individual components or as a group. This may lead to an enhancement of neoplastic induction, e.g. air pollution plus cigarette smoking, and confuse the development of etiological associations.

Systematically, the basis of epidemiological studies must rest upon the establishment of the frequency of disease in a given place and time. While morbidity data are of relatively recent origin, cancer mortality data have been collected for over a century. Problems of reliability (local and secular) of diagnosis are known to operate, nevertheless the relatively poor prognosis for cancer patients (except at certain sites) makes it less likely that such cases will be lost to epidemiologists.

Evaluation of Epidemiologic Methodologies

The methodologies utilized at present vary in their strength as well as their practicality.

Prospective.—The prospective method, if properly constructed, can minimize some problems to a certain extent, e.g. secular variation in diagnostic criteria. Cohort studies—subject to strict case registration control—minimize biases introduced by variations arising from losses to the study population in the course of time. Further, if morbidity can be determined in addition to mortality, the value of the study is enhanced, since it can be ascertained that people *did* or *did not* develop cancer rather than whether or not any individual died from this disease. Unfortunately, the major problem associated with the prospective study is one of expense (e.g. in establishing record systems, techniques of tracing individuals who have been lost to populations under study), plus the fact that too often fatal or potentially fatal effects must ensue to prove the point.

Retrospective.—In the retrospective study, in contrast to the prospective investigation, the last two practical objections are obviated to a considerable degree, though other problems take their place. It should be apparent that such studies depend upon the retrieval of records—collected for *other* purposes—of events occurring in the past, e.g. deaths, living habits, work exposures. These records are subject to uncontrollable variation of recorder origin in past time and place. Furthermore, even if patient or survivor interviews are obtained, the fact of the disease's occurrence per se will introduce biases by patients or survivors. Nevertheless, while this approach is less forceful than the prospective study, it has proved useful in many instances as an indicator of carcinogenic associations and as a preparatory step for more elaborate prospective study.

Combined.—A combination of the prospective and retrospective approach consists of constructing cohorts of workers believed to be at risk. They are compared with other workers in the same site, industry or plant who are believed to be at *no* excess risk. The use of life tables permit one to follow in time past, but in a prospective fashion, the fate of persons within such cohorts. Variation of a secular nature may be minimized and some of the cost element of the prospective study may be avoided. However, other problems associated with retrospective studies may still intrude. This approach has begun to be used only in the last ten to fifteen years.

In summary, all epidemiological studies have several defects in common. The most serious of these arises from the variability in the dose of carcinogen that an individual worker may encounter. Hence, unless the carcinogenic agent is moderately or extremely powerful, a small increase in cancer in excess of the natural *background incidence,* e.g. 5 to 10 percent, may not be detected. Furthermore, unless the carcinogen induces a characteristic tumor—and especially at relatively unusual anatomical site—the ease of deriving an association is minimized. Thirdly, because of the long latent periods of so many carcinogens, unless workers enter employment at an early age, the period of life during which occupational tumors appear coincides with the age at which most non-occupational tumors are found to appear. Finally, there is an impediment common to epidemiological investigations of any type in industry, namely, corporate fear of legal liability (both occupational and commercial) in the event that an association is demonstrated.

Examples of Well-Designed Epidemiological Investigations

As examples of epidemiological studies representative of the most well-developed design, the investigations of Doll, Case, and

Lloyd may be profitably reviewed. While any epidemiologist examining a colleague's study can and will find elements to criticize, these studies can be considered as a standard of comparison for others in the epidemiological category.

Despite the previously mentioned caveats, it is clear that well-constructed and controlled epidemiological studies have succeeded in demonstrating powerful associations between a cancer and specific agents found in the occupational environment. This should not imply that other types of evidence have no role in dealing with the problem at hand. Nevertheless, and with full recognition of the criteria that must be met, since epidemiological evidence is the most useful scientific information ethically available regarding occupational cancer risk for *man*, we regard it as a most persuasive argument for societal action.

    Prospective.—In this category, a classical study is that of Doll and co-workers (1965) of British gas workers. The investigation was carried out over a time span of 8 years and covered 26,856 (later cut to 11,499) men. There were 34 occupational categories developed from four Gas Board rolls; exposure severity was classified at four levels. The population was followed up annually. All men on the rolls had worked five years or more, and were between the age of 40 and 65. The diagnoses were established by review of death certificates and the causes classified according to the WHO 1957 revised list. Standardized rates were corrected for age and compared with similar rates for England and Wales. A 10 percent sample of the study population was randomly selected to ascertain smoking habits. To check the reliability of death certificate recovery a 10 percent sample of one Gas Board roll was taken, revealing no substantial loss. As regards losses due to job turnover, retirement, etc., only 0.4 percent of men on the rolls could not be traced.

    Retrospective.—The study of Case *et al.* (1954) represents a useful standard of performance for retrospective epidemiology. While this was a proportional mortality study, many of the shortcomings of such an approach were minimized. The exposed population was derived from company rolls, hospital records and death certificates of the geographical area. The problems associated with the effects of biases in the same geographical areas should apply in the control group. Because of the enlightened co-operation of industrial management the problems of dependence upon death-certificated occupational designations were obviated. This co-operation made categorization of specific job groupings within the industry accessible for evaluation of relative risks within these undertakings. As regards the control population, the delineation of death rates was soundly based statistically, appropriate age corrections being applied to all populations under study. Secular variation both in control and exposed populations was examined for multiple variables. The study might possibly have been improved by a more definitive cohort construction.

Combined.—The studies of Lloyd and co-workers (1969/70/71) represent an uncommonly well-executed example of the combined approach, i.e. a prospective study performed in retrospect. To avoid the biases introduced by comparing mortailty rates of industrial and non-industrial populations, the control group was drawn from workers in the same industry believed not to be exposed to the risks under study. Such risks could be clearly defined for 57,072 steel workers, since company rolls were freely available to the investigators. Extensive efforts to ascertain the fate of all workers leaving employment were especially effective, i.e. less than 0.2 percent of all workers could not be accounted for. Causes of death were ascertained from death certificates and coded according to the Seventh Revision of the International Statistical Classification (WHO). Using such complete data, it was possible to establish a cohort of exposed workers whose mortality experience could be compared with an industrially-based control population. Although these data represent events occurring in the past, this study design permits the investigator to follow in a prospective fashion the mortality experiences of those populations over a period of time.

Problems of Epidemiologic Evaluation

The problems encountered in the evaluation of occupational exposure to suspected carcinogens requires an understanding of the variable nature of work and production cycles. Such variability contributes significantly to the problems involved in elucidating dose-response relationships occurring in industry. Even though the basic question of the shape of the dose-response curve at its lower extent is open to discussion, nevertheless, qualitative and quantitative questions of dose are relevant to the delineation and understanding of industrial cancer. Since *dose* is a function of concentration and duration (Ct), we shall consider each of these two variables separately. As regards evaluation of the *quantity* of carcino-

genic exposure encountered in a workplace:such determinations—
even given optimum environmental monitoring capabilities—are
rarely accomplished *in toto*. An important reason for this paucity
of extensive work-exposure data is the periodicity of production
cycles—both over a long and short term. Frequently the atmospheric discharge from a process is a function of the type of apparatus used in production, ingredients, intermediates and end-pro-
ducts. Many of these will reflect economics, varying temporally to
meet variations in product requirements, availability of raw materials, or because of the age or modifications to production apparatus. In addition, engineering or technical personnel will frequently institute variations in ingredient mix, vessel temperature,
pressure or time cycle to achieve economic or product enhancement. Thus, while the reaction-steps for the production of a specific
chemical product may be generically similar between plants and
countries, these minor changes will introduce variation in the
quantity of chemicals encountered in each workplace. With wear
and tear of equipment, variations in maintenance practices will
markedly affect the possibility for and the quantity of incidental
chemical discharge in the working environment. Between plants—
and dependent upon age of equipment and availability of capital
for improvement—the extent of technical hygienic control will
vary. This source of variation may also reflect existent statutory
requirements for control, or labor union concerns; the degree to
which such statutes are enforced will affect the quantity of workplace contamination. Finally, in no plant will each of these factors
affecting the quantity of chemical exposure remain constant over
time. Accordingly, with this time-dependent ebb and flow, each
individual factor governing the quantitative aspects of worker
exposure will vary in time as well as from place to place.

Other approaches to estimation of dose have been utilized.
While the assessment of body burden by agents which enter the
body via the respiratory tract is amenable to quantitation by use of
standard atmospheric sampling techniques, those agents capable of
percutaneous absorption pose more difficult problems. Quantitative
estimates have been attempted by measurement of occupationally
encountered chemicals deposited upon gauze skin patches, in hand-
washing, as metabolites in body excreta, or as settled dust. How-

ever, these approaches for non-respiratory exposures are but gross quantitative measures of risk. Indeed, even for respiratory absorption (which is more accessible to quantitation) particle size, solubility and thus the extent of pulmonary uptake can vary as a function of any of the changes in production characteristics previously noted. Thus it should be apparent that even the optimum environmental evaluation represents an approximation.

Since dose is also a function of the duration of exposure, examination of this parameter requires estimation. Variations in production methods, equipment modifications, environmental controls, etc. noted previously will also obviously affect the duration (short term and long) as well as the severity of exposure. Furthermore, since production usually reflects economic supply and demand, processes may be only periodically operative. Records of production volumes are not usually retained over the period of time required for adequate study. Yet, more important than production variation, the movement of individual workers in or out of a specific work area cannot be determined with certainty but for the recent past. Between factories, designation of job titles vary, similar titles do not necessarily reflect similar exposures. Additionally, variations introduced by employee turnover, upgrading or mobility, etc. introduce intangible variables in any estimation of man-years of risk.

Quite aside from these questions of Ct determination, other *qualitative* parameters will determine carcinogenic exposure severity. From time to time, the nature of the raw materials will vary as to affect risk. Economic and other availability factors will determine the varying degrees of purity or the nature of contaminants associated with raw materials. The qualitative nature of intermediate reaction products is rarely known; these intermediates usually are not considered to have any economic or technical implication, hence there is no motivation for their characterization. The same problem applies to product residues as well as materials which remain in lines or reactors. (This problem may apply to a lesser degree in the future, since product contaminants may have important commercial ramifications dependent upon their ultimate use; e.g. for pharmaceuticals and fine chemicals, characterization of product contaminant is mandatory; for heavy chemicals, such considerations are at present commercially irrelevant.) The carcinogenic nature of chemical compounds may also vary because of changes in their chemical or physical state in the course of reactions due to solvent, diluents or vehicles used (see discussion of animal testing below), or the temperatures employed. All these will vary with time and place and will impede both environmental evaluation and design of experimental investigation which aims at reproduction of occupational exposure.

The question of the presence of impurities and contaminants is especially important when considering qualitative factors which impede epidemiological investigations. Contaminants present in starting materials, as well as product, usually reflect economically determined limitations on technology's application to the solution of impurity removal. That is, each redistillation, fractionation or eutectic separation of a mixture, while enhancing the possibility for separation of an impurity (isomeric or others), also increases price, especially as the degree of purity increases. Accordingly—and especially when dealing with the large volumes common to industrial usage—the grade (purity) of chemical used or produced will reflect such realities of cost structures. As an example of this question of *product-purity* one can readily cite the case of alpha-naphthylamine and the problem of removing its isomer, beta-naphthylamine. While purification of alpha can be readily achieved to allow a 4 to 5 percent beta contamination, to achieve a 1 percent beta content will increase the cost of such a product, while to obtain a product containing only 0.1 percent concentration level of beta will make such a product non-competitive for industrial usage (unless a compelling reason for using such a relatively more purified alpha-naphthylamine supervenes). This cost-dependent reality of contamination of alpha-naphthylamine with its beta isomer has impeded resolution of a highly relevant question in this area of industrial carcinogenesis: In view of beta's apparently high potency as a human carginogen, is the carcinogenic potency of alpha only apparent, or is it real; is alpha carcinogenic per se, or does it only appear so because of the beta isomer's presence in industrial grade alpha?

Unless these technical variations are understood and recognized by the investigator, assumptions as to comparability of data arising from different times or places may be patently erroneous. While recognition of these differences is crucial in comparing various populations at risk, such recognition and attempts at standardization of exposure risk serves to diminish population sizes and impedes the development of epidemiological associations.

Host-Biologic Variation

Evaluation of the nature of the occupational exposure is difficult; understanding of the biologic variables governing human response remains opaque. This will continue to present serious problems until our understanding of the biology of neoplastic response is improved (see above). Questions might theoretically exist regarding the role of biologic variations on *susceptibility* toward neoplastic alteration. The course of metabolic degradation or activation of a carcinogen depends upon genetic determinants; hence the manner in which a potential carcinogen acts will reflect variations in genetic pools that vary with time and place. While the genetic variations responsible for modifications of glucose-6-phosphate dehydrogenase or dibucaine number are well established, possibilities for similar genetically determined variations in metabolic handling of carcinogens, though not known, may exist. Thus, what *may* be weakly carcinogenic in one time, place or population, may not be equally so in another, or vice versa. Ultimately, such genetic pool variations may play a role in the determination of the *background noise level* of naturally occurring cancers, be these a result of purely genetic variation, if such exists, or response to environmental carcinogens. It should be recognized that at present the foregoing consideration of biological variations remains theoretical.

Host-General Environmental Variations

Man's dietary is usually determined by general environmental factors, e.g. economic and social. The variations encountered are as extensive as the human experience. It appears that diet plays some role in the induction of cancer. For instance, liver tumor induction by amino azo dyes is strongly but variably influenced by the level of riboflavin (Miller and Miller, 1953). Although animal models do suggest the reality of dietary factors, there is little clear-cut evidence that dietary constituents play a role in human carcinogenesis.

The existence of naturally occurring carcinogens has been clearly established. For instance, the well established hepatic carcinogenicity of senecio alkaloid has clear implications as regards human cancer occurrence. In addition, the association of the product of Aspergillus flavus, aflotoxin, and liver tumors in trout is clear. The relatively higher frequency rate of such cancers in Nigeria has been noted (Dunham and Bailar), while intake of groundnut-meal subject to mold-promoting conditions is known to be a part of the local dietary.

Other social habits associated with the quality of food intake may influence cancer occurrence. The extraordinary prevalence of the esophageal carcinoma in the Turkmen SSR (Dunham and Bailar) has been attributed by some to ingestion of highly-heated foods. A non-food intake of Swazi snuff, rich in nickel and chromium, has been recently demonstrated to be associated with a markedly increased incidence of maxillary antral carcinoma in the Bantu of South Africa (Baumslag *et al.*).

Finally, the universal usage of combustion products of various vegetable leaves plays an unconestable role in induction of cancer. The evidence at this time clearly defines a significantly enhanced risk of pulmonary carcinoma among heavy tobacco leaf smokers (USPHS 1964).

This association has already complicated our understanding of industrial carcinogenesis among asbestos workers. Selikoff *et al.* have clearly shown that risk of developing pulmonary cancers among such workers dramatically rises in proportion to daily cigarette consumption. Whether asbestos per se would cause the inductio of bronchiogenic carcinomic is probably not open to question in view of the ability to reproduce lung cancers in animals (Gross, *et al.* 1967). The same would undoubtedly be said of bladder tumors among smokers who have worked with beta-naphythylamine, viz. suggestions of an association between smoking and bladder tumors among the general population could affect to some degree the outcome of occupational exposure to beta.

In both these cases the role of smoking might be said to be additive; the question of whether it could be determinative of carcinogenesis probably does not apply among such workers. But the problem of the co-carcinogenic influence of smoking will become more important—as regards tipping the balance between producing or not producing a cancer—when we are faced with the weak industrial carcinogen. For while in such cases smoking may be causative, it could also be additive; conversely, a weak occupational carcinogen may potentiate the effect of cigarette smoking. In order to distinguish between causation and promotion in humans epidemiologic methods must be applied. Such studies will require large populations, and even if these are available will tax the power of this investigational method. Indeed, it is questionable whether sufficiently large industrial populations exposed to carcinogens can be developed except on national study bases, e.g. the asbestos studies of Selikoff, the studies of Case *et al.*, 1954.

While the probability is that such a dissection of cause and co-carcinogenic effect is probably not readily susceptible to clarification—and might even be considered academic, the implications for equitable adjudication of industrial cancer claims are not unreal. From a practical viewpoint, the common-law principle (United Kingdom, United States) that the employer accepts the worker *as he is* would appear to be one reasonable way out of this impasse.

Variations in Statistical Data

One of the basic problems in the utilization of human cancer experience data stems until recently from our incomplete knowledge of the prevalence or frequency of cancer in the general population. Without reliable statistics describing occurrence of cancer in the general population, one is left at a disadvantage when attempting to attribute an increased relative occurrence of neoplasia in an occupational group. Without a standardized frequency rate, one cannot determine what the expected rate for a tumor might be. While this defect has been minimized in certain nations with the establishment of cancer registries, their existence is less than universal. Where such do exist, it is possible to ascertain the existence of reasonable local variations in cancer incidence. While the importance of such geographically localized rates becomes of the utmost importance (e.g. see the study of Hill and Faning), even such use of mortality records suffers the problem common to all, i.e. they may be diluted or obscured by reporting variations introduced by physicians (local nosologic fashions notwithstanding attempts at standardized diagnoses!) or by simply physician or hospital inertia or indifference to registry requests. Certainly, while international co-operation in the development of nosologic and classification standards represents a beginning at resolution of these matters (see Histopathological Definition and Classification of Tumors, WHO, 1970), such systems rise or fall upon the levels of professional diagnostic capability and diligence in specificity of death reporting.

Still another problem relates to the size of a high-risk population available for study. Vouchsaving that one can define adequately a population at risk, such industrial groups usually turn out to be individually small in any one plant. Thus, when one looks for malignant events involving specific organs, e.g. the urinary bladder, one finds that the expected rates for such occurrences is quite small. This applies even for more common tumors, e.g. the expected number of lung tumors in the Bradford Hill and Faning study being 1.01 for 11 persons. While 11 individuals constitute a small population, the fact remains that the number of workers needed to produce relatively large volumes of chemicals in any one plant usually is quite small.

These facts lead the investigator towards the collection of statistics from several plants throughout an industry. In turn, one is then faced with all the variations connected with differences in work cycles of production methods, ingredients and mixes, etc. discussed above. Finally, among studies of multiple plant sites, the thorough investigator should attempt to determine the prevalence of malignant diseases based upon local frequency of that pathological process. This has, in fact, infrequently been essayed.

Another serious problem associated with the epidemiological approach to industrial disease studies stems from losses of individuals from the population at risk. This is especially pertinent in occupational cancer because of this disease's long latent period. Persons who have longevity sufficient to receive sickness and health benefits from an employer may be relatively readily traced through such records even after they have left employment. However, the young short-term worker who had a relatively short exposure (e.g. 1-5 years) is not traceable through his former employer's records after 10 to 20 years, yet given expected latent periods, this *lost case* introduces unfortunate bias. In nations with national health and sickness benefit programs many such cases can be found, their attribution to a specific type of employment may well require interfacing several different record systems, e.g. one in the Ministry of Labor, the other in a national social security agency. Parenthetically, the interesting approach of Mancuso *et al* utilizing Social Security Administration records may conflict with the wish of discouraging the use of such data. There are fears that access will establish precedents likely to impair their confidentiality and to allow the misuse of these records.

Finally, other legal implications involved in a reporting process may vitiate the values of such systems. Where sickness or death benefits may place liability upon an employer or insurance company, attribution of cancer deaths to work may be denied by such parties. The ultimate disposition of such claims may be dependent in the end upon non-medical or administrative adjudications of such questions. Conversely, because extra benefits may accrue because of work connected neoplasia, a tendency for a local over-attribution can further militate against the use of these records.

Case studies and Reports

In contrast to the well-ordered systematic epidemiological study, we find the clinical case series or report. Since such observations are collected with varying degrees of concern for many important contributory variables, the value of such data is compromised. Reports may vary from the collection of cases which appear to cluster about one industrial group or geographical area, down to the individual clinical case report. Though all degrees between these extremes may obtain, all such studies suffer from several disadvantages, viz., uncontrolled observer variation and an inadequate or absent statistical base.

Concerning the variation inherent in case observations, a primary difficulty resides in the lack of diagnostic criteria standardization. This is frequently compounded by an inability on the part of clinicians to obtain adequate work or agent exposure histories, as well as deficiencies in their follow-up of case reports. The statistical foundations of this category of data are weak, since there may be little or no population basis upon which to found allegations of an unusual frequency of occurrence. Also absent are comparisons of expected rates for all cancers studied in that time or place. Accordingly, while aggregates or case series reports cannot be ignored, they should at best only be considered as collateral data inputs.

Nevertheless, consideration of their possible merit suggests that if experimental evidence of cargenosis develops, individual case reports take on a new meaning in the assessment of carcinogenicity. The use of such data to butress the case for carcinogenicity is inadequate, however, unless clustering is prominent and/or the precise nature of the carcinogenic contact can be identified.

PROBLEMS IN CONNECTING EXPERIMENTAL CARCINOGENESIS WITH OCCUPATIONAL CANCER

Choice of Species and Strain of Experimental Animals

There appears to be considerable variation in the ability of an individual compound to incite tumors when applied to various species. For example, while rabbits—relative to mice and rats—appear refractory to subcutaneous induction of skin tumors by the polycyclic hydrocarbons, this generalization fails if cotton-tail rabbits are injected with 20-methylcholanthrene (Syverton *et al.*); the rabbit is refractory to induction of liver tumors by azo compounds, while the mouse is susceptible to such tumor induction but not to the same degree as the rat. By contrast, the mouse skin is more susceptible to action of polycyclic hydro-carbons than is the rat. The matter of the choice of experimental species was proven to be critical as regards the experimental reproduction of the human bladder lesion found in the dye-staff industry and the resolution of the 2-naphthylamine question; until the dog was used, reproduction of this tumor could be achieved only with difficulty.

Another complication of the species problem is the question of strain variation occurring within a species. Such complication, especially from the point of view of the epidemiologist, is more apparent than real. In testing an unknown chemical for carcinogenic capacity, a random-bred stock gives a wider diversity of genetic line and thus a larger probability for detecting neoplastic potentials. Furthermore, such random-bred populations more clearly mimic the breeding characteristics of humans. On the other hand, for the investigator, the availability of inbred lines provides several advantages. For one reason, the incidence of tumors in such lines can be more consistently predicted within a strain; for another, in the study of structure-function relationship for a homologous group of chemicals, one is more likely to obtain reproducible and reliable results within such inbred lines. Thus, both random and inbred strains have their uses and limitations; how to take advantage of breeding variables appears more manageable than is the question of species choice.

Dosage and Scheduling Problems in Experimental Design

Because of variations due to species, dosage scheduling (duration, amount, frequency), routes of administration, criterion of response and use (intended or otherwise) of modifiers, the experimentalist is faced with serious questions in the design of tests for carcinogenicity. Concerning the *quantity* of chemicals to be administered: the experimentalist obtains the maximum potential for detection of tumorogenic activity by use of a maximum dose consistent with long-term longevity of his animals. Two problems attach themselves to this practice: increasing dose beyond a certain point may decrease tumor yield (Terracini *et al.*) and the relevance to human exposure has been considered by some to be somewhat attenuated. Further, at the high dose level, alteration of physiologic status may enhance neoplasia by indirect mechanisms (e.g. enhanced quantity of reparative hyperplasia). While the former question can be met by increasing the *range* of dose levels (and accordingly cost in time and resources) the latter requires another answer. Contrariwise, questions relating to the effect of promoting agents (e.g. Croton oil, certain Tween, Spans), recognized or not, may obfuscate the reality of the lower end of the dose response curve.

Closely related to dose consideration are questions of determining test population size required for screening of carcinogenic potential. One of the most clear-cut justifications for a large dose is a forcing of the issue of "carcinogenic or not?" This becomes particularly pertinent in the case of weak carcinogens, since the alternative for detection of a weak carcinogen would be the use of a very large population. Yet even increasing the population size to such proportions may still produce a small yield, e.g. as in the case of a 5 percent incidence level for a weak carcinogen, a yield most prudent experimentalists would consider as open to question. Accordingly, rather than hoping to detect low potency carcinogens by the use of an inordinately large population, the choice of population size should be governed by use of more precise statements of confidence limits desired, plus use of large doses (v.s.).

Beyond the question of quantity is the matter of frequency of dosing. While earlier evidence suggested that the total size of carcinogen required to bring about 100 percent skin tumor incidence varies inversely with length of time between administration (Cramer and Stowell), later treatments of similar data have clarified this question. Wynder *et al.* have clearly demonstrated that small carcinogenic doses are indeed quantitatively additive, regardless of schedule. Some reservations to this position can be stated: the time between dosing should not be sufficiently large as to permit cell *recovery*.

Since the scheduling of doses is important, another facet of this question concerns the period of testing and observation. Earlier experiments have failed to detect carcinogenic potentials when chemicals were tested for relative short periods of time (days or a few months). As a general rule, testing should cover a period of 1/3 to 1/2 of a life span, though Heuper recommends that the whole life span be subjected to testing in species having less than five years longevity. Because of a *manageable* life span, the rat has been used in preference to other animals, e.g. the dog. The problem inherent in this approach to carcinogenic screening is well illustrated by the difficulties encountered in the induction of bladder tumors with beta naphtylamine in species other than the dog. Consequently, such facts once more point to the necessity of the use of multiple species—although the cost and inconvenience increases; the possible traps when convenience governs our choices of species have been self-evident.

Choice of Sex and Age of Experimental Animals

Related to these questions are those regarding the age and sex of animal to be tested. The young adult age would be more analogous to occupationally exposed groups; however, some carcinogens appear to be particularly active in the developing pre- and neo-natal brain and central nervous system. An extensive recent literature, indicating the carcinogenic and teratogenic potential of nitroso compounds administred to pregnant rats, suggests that low doses of such compounds may exert severe effects such as general malformations as well as subsequent cancers in the offspring (Napalkov and Alexandrov; Rice). That such effects have human parallels has been suggested also by the reports of oestrogenic agents administered to pregnant humans which have resulted in tumors of the offspring (Anon, 1971; Greenwald, *et al*).

Such experimental results have obvious implications as concerns the exposure of pregnant women in the course of their work to agents—the present spectrum of which is unknown—which may have such severe teratogenic and tumorogenic effects.

Route and Mode of Dosing

Especially pertinent to the protection of workers against carcinogenic agents are considerations of the portal of entry of such materials, especially in relation to experimental investigations. Whereas most general investigations of chemical carcinogenicity do not utilize the respiratory portal entry, this route represents an extremely common avenue for occupational uptake. While the relevance of subcutaneous implantation of polymers and other chemicals to the occupational exposure is highly questionable, such is not necessarily the case in the experimentalist's use of other portals for other substances.

As regards mimicking the respiratory portal of entry, (and where problems do not involve local pulmonary carcinogenesis) whichever route is utilized experimentally (respiratory *or* parenteral) the end result may be essentially the same, i.e. absorption of the agent for systematic distribution and specific organ metabolic activation. This also applies to a degree as regards the relationship of oral administration and occupational exposure, though some quantitative modifications of results may stem from variations induced by, e.g. degree of gastrointestinal absorption or chemical alteration. Certainly the reality of occupational exposure—regardless of engineering control—includes inadvertent oral intake or unconsicious swallowing of the products of pulmonary clearance. In view of the relatively frequent failure to induce pulmonary tumors with known lung carcinogens, testing solely of that portal of entry may fail to detect presently unsuspected carcinogenic potentialities for agents that may act at the pulmonary locus.

Failures to chemically reproduce tumors that are known to occur in humans have necessitated other design strategies. For example, the beta-napthylamine bladder tumor was reproduced by feeding only with difficulty until the dog was used. In the face of the reality of the workplace, not to have attempted bladder implants in rodents, especially of the putative human metabolites, would have been puristically unreasonable in determining which component of the aniline mixture was carcinogenic. For another reason, such strategies offer a ready opportunity for the study of morphology and pathology of such tumor and the biochemistry of such compounds. However, the role of concretions of bladder following implantation per se in inducing bladder tumors should be recognized (Weil et al), especially in testing of low potency carcinogens. In essence, some degree of judgment must be employed regarding relevance of experimental routes of administration to occupational realities. How one regards experiments utilizing subcutaneous implants of relatively inert polymers or similar placement of metallic compounds under a high degree of suspicion of carcinogenicity is susceptible to differing possibilities. By contrast, experiments using high doses of chemicals which may or may not represent the human metabolite, and which cause weak carcinogenic response, means one thing in screening experiments designed to test a material for human consumption and quite another for working populations. It is sufficient to say that an almost endless variety of insoluble materials placed in tissues will cause subsequent tissue response and powerful carcinogenic alterations even after these materials are removed. While one would be foolhardy to apply results at their face value to the occupational mileau, one can not nevertheless totally reject such experimental results. Materials which are capable of inciting tumors, regardless of circumstances of administration, cannot be totally disregarded because their behavior falls within a general category of responses to foreign materials implanted in tissues. How one regards such data will be ultimately determined by considerations which are relevant to the mode of use or nature of exposure to such agents.

Solvent or Vehicles used in an Experiment

Such materials may have a considerable effect upon the results of cancer induction. Thus any comparison of various experimental reports requires close scrutiny of agents used as carcinogen solvents or vehicles. Such consideration revolves about questions of carcinogenicity of these carriers, e.g. the co- or the carcinogenicity of cholesterol (Weil-Malherbe and Dickens), the inhibition or enhancement of tumor formation because the variations in phospholipid content of vehicles (ibid.), the physical binding properties which alter rates of release of agents to tissues (Strait, *et al.*) or the effect of some purines which enhance solubilisation of a carcinogen leading to an inhibitory effect upon tumors induction (Brock). All of these factors require careful evaluation. Such details could obscure applicability of laboratory data to occupational exposures, particularly where mixed carcinogen-solvent combinations occurred in the workplace. Such solvent effects designed to enhance tumor production must be understood to represent means to the end such as are achieved by use of high doses of agents; accordingly applicability to the workplace should be regarded in the light of these experimental enhancement techniques.

Closely related to dosing considerations is the question of the purity of a compound under animal test. Advances in analytical methodologies have enhanced potentials for detection of compounds in the picogram, or lower, range. Certainly given the problems of organic synthesis and separation, removal of trace contaminants at such levels of detection becomes increasingly more difficult. This problem may be especially important experimentally when considering compounds of purported low carcinogenicity. Furthermore, detection, and possible quantitation, of contaminants (even at the 10^{-12} to 10^{-15} molar concentration) is similarly pertinent in testing commercial products, since impurities here are relevant in assuring public safety.

Animal Diet and Care Variations

It is a general maxim that the general health of experimental animals must be relatively normal if experimented reproducibility is expected. The effect of dietary constituents upon carcinogenesis has been clearly seen (v.s. effects of riboflavin deficiency). The particular requirements of specific species must be anticipated if normal growth curves are to be obtained. While such details of dietary regimen may be apparent, they also may be in some regards more apparent than real.

The reliability of the supplier (or the sophistication of the experimenter) are often the only barriers between spurious effects induced by stilbesterol contaminated feeds, or the absence of over-heating of lipid constituents in manufacture (and the production of co- or carcinogens). Mold contamination of feed may introduce the possibility of highly toxic or hepatocarcinogenic but inadvertant additives. The details of animal care, cage construction, avoidance of cross or recontamination, the use of pesticides for vermin control—all require documentation. Inadequacies of space, low quality of animal care, or construction and sanitation of animal care facilities all may adversely affect the results of experiment. Despite the possible variations in experimental response engendered by such problems, such important details are usually inapparent or must be assumed in research reports.

Diagnostic Criteria and Evaluation of Carcinogenic Potency

The accessibility of a tumor to inspection will markedly affect our ability to measure its course of development. Thus while the presence of skin and ear-duct tumors can be detected in their early stages sufficient to quantitatively assess carcinogenicity in terms of dose or latency (Druckrey, 1962) palpatory evaluation of abdominal tumor may not be similarly satisfactory. Inspection even of superficial tumors poses problems of comparability between reports, e.g. diagnostic criteria for standardizing beginning points of tumors, size, duration or persistence. The care and adequacy of exploratory laparotomy, the familiarity of the pathologist with the normal anatomy of the experimental animal, will all determine the reliability of evaluation. These factors in the assessment of carcinogenesis are especially relevant in attempting to compare reports from several laboratory groups.

Two variables largely express carcinogenic activity of a compound. The *latent period* is defined as the time interval between first dosing and the appearance of the first tumor in the test group. Since this period is generally inversely proportional to the dose, the latent period is valid experimentally only for a given dosage. The other variable expressing carcinogenic potential is *tumor incidence*, defined as a proportion of surviving animals bearing tumors. What constitutes the total effective population may be open to contention; accordingly, the definition of population at risk frequently is reported in terms of the condition of the individual experiment. Utilizing both parameters of response, i.e. latent period and tumor incidence, numerous investigators have attempted quantitative evaluation of the dose-response relationship in studying induced skin tumors. Linear relationships between dose and incidence and/or latency (Bryan and Shimkin, 1942-43; Druckrey *et al*, 1962) have suggested the existence of a threshold for carcinogenic response. It should be emphasized that these viewpoints depend upon the mathematical validity of the probit analyses utilized and the low dose extrapolations of these investigators; this procedure is believed by some investigators to be open to question. It is this group's viewpoint that downward extrapolation of data along a linear plot of a probit analysis is invalid since it goes beyond the available data. By contrast, in the hands of other investigators, quantitative approaches to the testing of skin carcinogenic potencies has demonstrated a relatively more regular relationship between latency period and dose, while relationships between incidence and dose are considerably less consistent. This latter poor association probably stems from difficulties in quantitative application of skin doses (see Horton, *et al*.) and has undoubtedly been aggravated by variations introduced in use of solvents (Horton and Denman), periodicity of application, etc.

Further complicating studies of neoplastic potentiality is the question of the effects of discontinuous applications. While earlier work of Cramer and Stowell indicating an increase in dose was required if the interval between doses was increased, re-examination of that data (Arcos, Argus and Wolf) and the report of Wynder *et al.* have more clearly indicated that small carcinogenic doses are additive, as long as the dose-free interval is not sufficiently protracted to permit cell *repair* to take place.

There have been numerous attempts made to grade carcinogenic potency based upon tumor incidence, latent period or the time required to induce tumors in 50 percent of animals. While problems such as dose-concentration variations, solvents, vehicles, or schedules are susceptible to standardization, the determination of maximum effective dose for most carcinogens remains to be made. That is, dose increases beyond such a maximum may well lead to decreased incidence (Terracini *et al.*), so that standardized determinations of maximum effective doses would be required to make such grading indices truly quantitative.

Extrapolation of Animal Data to Man

Intrinsic to all the foregoing has been an unstated but omnipresent concern, i.e. how do we judiciously relate animal experiments to human societal needs and requirements. Unfortunately, there are few, if any principles which provide a consistent resolving capacity for answering this question; critical judgments are always required. In general, where tumors are similar morphologically and occur in the same organ as in man, such findings are obviously highly relevant. However, it should be emphasized that this approach has neither absolute predictive or preventive value; further, in view of our inability to induce arsenical tumors in animals and the suggestive evidence that such occur in man, might not a converse situation cause us to miss potential carcinogens of human significance if we depended upon animal experimentation? In essence, our problem in use of experimental data may be stated: given the relative weakness of the epidemiological method to detect low order tumor incidence increases, positive evidence of animal carcinogenicity also can do much to answer questions of human risk although some limitations should be recognized accordingly. The experimentalist can point the way to further epidemiological investigation, or serve to warn prior to undertaking commercial production of a chemical.

Another criterion supposedly enhancing relevance is phylogenetic proximity. By this measure, the most meaningful test species should be primates. Yet long-term attempts at induction of epithelial carcinogenesis by hydrocarbons in the Rhesus (Pfeiffer and Allen) have been unsuccessful. Such stands in contrast to successful experimental applications utilizing lower animals, e.g. rodent skin, to produce tumors similar to those seen in exposed workers.

Ironically, it is becoming clear that we can more judiciously state some *principles* concerning what does *not* constitute relevance for man. Induction of sarcomas following subcutaneous implantation of various non-specific materials, e.g. plastics, metal, films, suggest that physical or chemical variables peculiar to that mode of administration may precipitate such tumors. Further, species or strains in which the control incidence of a tumor is of high frequency also have diminished importance to man. The work of Clayson *et al.* and the report of Weil *et al.* place serious question upon bladder implant for the induction of tumors, especially when involving compounds of low carcinogenic potency. It appears that the physical presence of some materials in the urinary bladder act as mechanical irritants and promote miotic activity of the bladder epithelium. Finally, tissues which commonly are associated with viral tumors, e.g. leukemia and lymphomas, should be considered cautiously because of non-specific or accidental complicating factors (Clayson). The middle ground between these two *extreme* limits finds relevance a subject of contention. Disregarding animal evidence and dependency on human demonstration of carcinogenicity carries the risks inherent in the weaknesses of the epidemiologic method. Thus, a tumor having 5 percent incidence is considered experimentally as a weak carcinogen, but will cause 50 cases in a population of 1,000 individuals. In view of the fact that few industrial populations at risk of this size can be readily aggregated, and because there is little that biologically distinguished such occupationally induced tumors from the usual *background noise-level* of cancers, what is a weak carcinogen to the researcher may become a serious problem to the occupational health specialist. Therefore, animal data—even at high dose levels—cannot be ignored unless there is a very strong body of evidence such as to clearly, unequivocally deny even low carcinogenic potential; unfortunately, in most cases such evidence is not readily adduced. Because the worker in industry absorbs carcinogens mainly through the respiratory tract or by way of skin contact, experiments utilizing other portals of entry carry only somewhat less weight, as regards human relevance in industry. If it can be shown that a chemical can be absorbed via these portals, injection studies immediately assume greater significance.

Complicating the entire question of how one regards experimental data is the observation of the additive nature of small doses of carcinogens, even though such may be of differing charcateristics or nature. Hence, considering multiple additive effects of the same or different compounds, we begin to perceive a setting which might be quite similar to reality: an environment potentially composed of an almost unlimited combination of multiple agents. It has been suggested that carcinogenic hazard decreases—but never completely disappears—with diminishing dose.

In summarizing experimental modes, clearly the elucidation of the chemical nature of carcinogenic or polycyclic hydrocarbons and azo dyes has rapidly progressed, thanks to such approaches. At first, it was the hope of researchers that by testing a large and diverse group of chemical classes, recognition of a common specific molecular configuration of characteristic would point the way to better understanding of the cellular events leading to cancer. Except for the fact that grossly the reactive form of most carcinogens apparently contain electron deficient atoms (Miller & Miller, 1971) little other commonality is discerible. Never-the-less, such studies have produced useful information in coping with industrial cancer hazards. In addition, they have enhanced the possibility of primary prevention (i.e. prevention of occurrence) by giving advance warning of carcinogenic potentials of various products or materials (e.g. 2-acetylaminofluorene, a insecticide which was never put into production on the basis of tumor induction in rats). At the same time as there has been a burgeoning diversity of chemicals developed there has also been a coincidental increase in the number of chemicals which individually are reported as having carcinogenic properties. The use of animal tests should—theoretically—resolve two pertinent questions of societal choice.

1) At what point do we cease investing resources in development and production of a chemical because of a finding of carcinogenic capacity under a variety of circumstances, relevant and possibly relevant?

2) What degree of human risk (or workers, of society) is per-

missible, consistent with the achievement of which social needs are satisfied by a compound under consideration? (e.g. use of a pesticide of questionable carcinogenicity in an area of high malaria prevalence.

However, before one looks to the use of animal studies in order to answer these questions, a thorough understanding of the problems inherent in such testing procedures should serve to place into a proper perspective their uses and limitations. In the light of the present state of epidemiologic or experimentally derived knowledge this might lead one to the position that can be stated as follows: in the real world, if there is to be absolute control, evidence a this time indicates that protection cannot be provided at present, by threshold limits for carcinogenic agents. From all these foregoing considerations, it would appear that while disregarding any part of the laboratory evidence in regard to human risk is unwarranted, some operational, pragmatic approaches to coping with carcinogenic risk in industry must be developed. Indeed, biological evidence does suggest a wide spectrum of carcinogenic potency; similarly industrial experience supports this contention, e.g. for chromates and benzene. Therefore, because carcinogenic considerations in the industrial setting are not purely a function of the biological carcinogenic potencies per se (as discussed in the foregoing) an examination of the possible modes of control and of industrial experience in coping with occupational carcinogens should be taken into consideration (see page 66).

Chapter II

INDUSTRIAL AGENTS ASSOCIATED WITH HUMAN CARCINOGENIC RISK

EVALUATION OF EVIDENCE OF OCCUPATIONAL CARCINOGENESIS

Rationale for Hierarchy of Biological Proofs

THE PRECEDING CHAPTER has dwelt at length upon problems inherent in the use of experimental and epidemiological methods for adducing proof of human carcinogenicity. There we attempted to point out some of the problems regarding the utility of the experimental approach in the elucidation of the problem of human cancer.

Because we are dealing primarily wih the prevention of occupational cancer, our concern is perforce with the effects of carcinogenic agents upon human health. Accordingly, it should be apparent that since the epidemiological method utilizes human experience, the relevance of this approach is self-evident. While one would thus be pre-disposed to place great emphasis upon such proofs of carcinogenicity, critical assessment of the practical capabilities which the epidemiological method might bring to bear upon the problem is appropriate. It is within this context that any classification of carcinogenic potential has to be placed.

PROPOSED CLASSIFICATION OF BIOLOGICAL EVIDENCE FOR OCCUPATIONAL CARCINOGENESIS

General Principles—From the outset it should be clearly stated that the purpose of this classification is to rank order the weight

TABLE I

BIOLOGICAL EVIDENCE FOR OCCUPATIONAL
CARCINOGENIC POTENTIAL

Carcinogenic Potential for Man		Carcinogen	
		Chemical Compound or Element	Uncharacterized or Contaminated Mixtures
GROUP I- DEFINITELY CARCINOGENIC	*Type of evidence* Epidemiological + Experimental	beta-naphthylamine 4-aminodiphenyl chromium nickel benzidine	mineral derived tars, pitches, oils, asbestos
	Epidemiological	arsenic mustard gas	haematite
GROUP II- PROBABLY CARCINOGENIC	Epidemiological Associated with other carcinogens + Experimental	4-nitrobiphenyl alpha-naphthylamine	auramine magenta
	Experimental Cases?	beryllium	
	Cases only	benzene	
GROUP III- PRESUMABLY CARCINOGENIC	Animal experiments only	nitrosoamines, e.g. N-nitrosodimethylamine alkylating agents (with exception of mustard gas, dichlorobenzidine O-tolidine dianisidine	

of the evidence for occupational carcinogenicity among a group of materials or agents that are or could be found in the working environment. Biological evidence within our context refers to the broad spectrum of information including clinical, epidemiological and experimental data. In the light of the problems encountered in extrapolating animal-derived data to human needs, human experience is given more weight here than experimental evidence alone.

For reasons to be discussed later (see section on Control), the classification does not imply any ordering or priority for application of control measures for the prevention of occupational cancer. In addition, those categories must not be taken to imply an ordering of relative degrees of carcinogenic potency per se, since several of the compounds in Group III considered to be *presumably carcinogenic* are of a uniformly high oncogenic potency in animals. However, because of the orientation of this classification toward human occupational risk, absence of essential human experience with these Group III materials prevents our making a more definite statement regarding human carcinogenicity. This position should not be considered as minimizing the strong presumption that such agents would also be highly carcinogenic in the event that man-contact were to occur.

Furthermore, this classification should not be taken to indicate relative levels of carcinogenic ordering *even within grades.* For example, where experimentation presents design problems for benzidine induction of bladder tumors in animals, the strength of the epidemiological evidence for that compound's cancer potential in man leaves no more room for doubt of its potency than in the case, for example, of beta-naphthylamine (BNA). Conversely, as regards the chromates, epidemiological plus a single report of experimental induction (Laskin *et al.*) place chromates at the same level as benzidine in this evidentiary classification, even though it appears that the various salts and oxides of this element are less carcinogenic than benzidine.

Definition of Terms

Carcinogenic Potential for Man

GROUP I—DEFINITELY CARCINOGENIC. In this category are agents for which the evidence is extremely strong as regards human risk; they must be considered as having caused occupational cancer on the basis indicated under "Type of Evidence" (See Table I).

Epidemiological evidence as used here implies a reasonable meeting of the criteria for valid population-size, basis of comparison and collection techniques, standarization of diagnosis and statistical analytical methodologies; in addition, the factors of age, sex, etc., discussed previously must be considered and appropriate adjustments made.

Animal experimentation at this level implies that the morphology and organ locus of the experimental tumor is analogous to that found in man. The material should have been administered in such a fashion that its carcinogenic action occurs or is made to occur at the organ or site analogous to human cases (e.g. appropriate non-irritant bladder implant of human aromatic amine metabolites).

The doses employed to produce malignancies must be understood in terms of that optimally necessary to induce measurable responses (see previous discussion); a large-sized dose does not necessarily vitiate the applicability of such data to man who may encounter the material over a working life span.

GROUP II—PROBABLY CARCINOGENIC. In this category are agents for which evidence is relatively less incriminatory upon the basis of available information as compared to the preceding category. One group, because it may in the course of its manufacture be so intimately associated with carcinogens, is listed here, since its uncontrolled use per se carries ill-defined but probably excessive risk of causing human cancer. Carcinogenesis among such compounds may be due to their contamination—even by low concentrations—by the potent carcinogens with which they have been associated; however the evidence may be quite strong regarding inherent carcinogenesis of such compounds, e.g. 4-nitrobiphenyl. Materials which are listed in this Group on the basis of case reports are so considered because such data do not readily meet the criteria required of epidemiological investigations. Case reports in this context may be of an extensive or sporadic nature.

GROUP III—PRESUMABLY CARCINOGENIC. In this Group are a large number of chemicals, many of which have been studied by the experimental method but for which—with one exception i.e., mustard gas—no human carcinogenic data exists. The absence of such data may arise from the infrequency or absolute absence of industrial experience, or because populations at risk are too small to yield carcinogenic data basis, or because no investigations of human groups possibly exposed have been undertaken.

INDIVIDUAL CARCINOGENS

Chemical Compounds or Elements

In this category are compounds whose chemical nature can be clearly defined and characterized. In addition, included here are the specific elements which have been associated with carcinogenic potentials in the form of their various salts, oxides or complexes. It is not necessarily deduced that these *elements* are carcinogenic per se; in most cases precisely which form (s) is carcinogenic is not known.

Group I—Definitely Carcinogenic for Man
Epidemiological and Experimental Evidence

Beta-Naphthylamine (BNA)

EPIDEMIOLOGICAL EVIDENCE. Case and co-workers (1954) have demonstrated beyond question the association of this compound with human bladder tumors. The attack rate among exposed workers was extremely high (sixty-one times that of the general population) and involved workers at multiple stages of BNA manufacture as well as users of the product. While exposure in the remote past (prior to 1940) may have been more severe than later, because of the high attack rate and difficulties in control at multiple points in synthesis and in use, safe manufacture appears to be extremely difficult. For details of this study, see page 11. Critically, this study represents one of the better efforts in occupational cancer epidemiology, with the investigators extending the retrospective approach to its fullest, but not beyond.

EXPERIMENTAL EVIDENCE. Using the commercially available product, bladder tumors were reproduced in dogs (Hueper, Wiley and Wolfe). Because of differences in metabolic products these tumors could not be reproduced in other species until the human metabolite, 2-amino-1-naphthal, was incorporated in paraffin wax pellets for bladder implant in mice (Bonzer, Clayson and Jull, 1951).

USES AND OCCURRENCE. Primarily BNA is used in the production of dyes, coupling with diazotized bases as the end product of azo dyes. Small amounts of alpha- (as well as the beta-) isomer have been utilized as rubber vulcanization accelerators, as well as with xylidines and toluidines for ore flotation. As formyl and glycine derivatives, it has been used for rubber preservation as well as in the tanning industry.

COMMENTS. The carcinogenicity of BNA for man evidently leaves room for little question. The epidemiological study of Case *et al.* (1954) essentially constitutes a standard against which other retrospective studies can be compared. It is also pertinent to point out that while its carcinogenicity for man is accepted by all authorities, the reproduction of the urinary bladder tumor required considerable effort after many unsuccessful years of attempts.

4-Aminobiphenyl (4-AB)

EPIDEMIOLOGICAL EVIDENCE. On the basis of the series of Melick *et al.* (1955) and a follow-up of this group of exposed workers (Melamed *et al.*) handling commercial 4-AB, it can be clearly stated that this compound appears to be carcinogenic for man. The more recent follow-up (Melick, 1971) indicated a total work force of 315 persons exposed to this material, among whom 53 bladder tumors have been found.

EXPERIMENTAL EVIDENCE. Three bladder tumors have been found in 33 mice fed this chemical (Clayson *et al*, 1967) in addition to a significantly higher incidence of hepatomas in this species.

Out of 7 rats orally given commercial 4-AB, 1 papilloma and 3 cancers were found (Bonser, 1962). Various doses ranging as low as 1 mg/kg body weight have been administered to dogs, producing 7 carcinomas and 2 bladder papillomatoses in a total of 10 dogs (Walpole *et al.*, 1954, Deichmann *et al.*, 1958a, 1965).

USES AND OCCURRENCE. This compound was not manufactured on an industrial scale until 1938, when it was introduced in the USA as a rubber anti-oxidant. However, with the discovery of this material's carcinogenicity, production ceased and manufacture was never taken up elsewhere. Aside from this use the compound was present in *bottoms* of aniline stills at least during the nineteenth century, and may still be present (0.005 to 0.01 %) as a contaminant in the condensation synthesis of diphenylamine (Stagg and Reed).

COMMENT. In view of the human evidence, and a relatively high degree of carcinogenicity in several species, this compound would appear to have a strong evidentiary base for carcinogenicity to man.

Benzidine

EPIDEMIOLOGICAL EVIDENCE. The work of Case *et al.* (1954) has clearly shown this material to be carcinogenic for man. Workers in chemical factories exposed to benzidine, with or without aniline, were at fourteen-fold greater risk of developing bladder tumors as compared with an age-adjusted sub-population drawn from all males of England and Wales. The spectrum of workers incurring risk appears to extend through several stages of production (foremen, processmen, pressmen, filtermen, laborers, stillmen) and use, although the risk was not as extensively encountered as with BNA. By contrast with BNA, cases of bladder tumors are relatively less frequent among users, except for those engaged in processing the material for other uses.

The epidemiological study of Case was the same as cited for BNA, and has the same strengths.

Mancuso and El-Attar (1967) have confirmed the 1954 study of Case *et al.*, utilizing a retrospective method which achieved some of the elements of the prospective method; this was accomplished by retrospective construction of cohorts whose mortality could be followed over a twenty-five year period. While company rolls made possible the assignment of individuals to exposed and non-exposed categories, no other exposure data was available. Proportional mortalities were determined upon a bases of similar age-corrected mortalities expected in the same geographical area. In addition, an internal control made up of ostenibly *non-exposed* employees was utilized. This study revealed a significantly elevated risk of bladder and pancreatic cancers; it also indicated a relatively higher risk of cancer among workers handling BNA than was the case for those handling benzidine only. Hospital record follow-up indicated the usual under-reporting of neoplasia.

EXPERIMENTAL EVIDENCE. Bladder tumors have been induced only in dogs after long periods of relatively high dosages of 200 and 300 mg/day (Spitz as quoted by Bonzer *et al.*, 1956). It should be noted that while only three of seven dogs administred benzidine survived to manifest tumors after an extremely long latent period (seven to ten years), no control dogs were simultaneously studied.

The fact should be noted that experimental administration of benzidine produced tumors at multiple sites of various species: hepatomas and cymbel tumors in rats (Spitz *et al.*, 1950); hepatomas in mice (Bonser *et al*, 1956); and hamsters (Sellakumar *et al.*). These observations reinforce the need for considering this compound as carcinogenic. Even though bladder tumors per se have been induced with difficulty (see page 37), the loci of degradative enzymatic action—a function of the specific species in question—determines the organ at risk of neoplasia. Thus if multiple species developed tumors, though at different sites, any compound responsible for such alterations cannot be regarded lightly. Greater credence is given to this postion by the strength of the human data in the case of benzidine, i.e. it is well established that human risk exists; accordingly the difficulty with which experimental bladder tumors are produced is minimized by the evidence of multiple specie and site carcinogenesis. While experimental bladder tumor induction provides the strongest evidence for a similar risk in man, such multi-site and animal evidence cannot be ignored with impunity. Indeed, if one could definitely determine the active metabolite in man, properly designed experiments might minimize this problem of experimental induction (cf. Bonser, Clayson and Jull, 1951, for BNA).

Uses and Occurrence. Rubber hardener, *security* papers, azo dye intermediates, medical reagents.

Comments. The evidence for the carcinogenicity of benzidine is quite clear epidemiologically and incrimitative experimentally. As previously noted, the studies upon which we base this implication of carcinogenicity in man are probably the most direct ethical means for making such an ascertainment. The study populations were adequate in size, and had few losses from the rolls (Case *et al.*, 1954) because of the co-operation of the employers and the steps taken by the investigators to follow up such rolls. The occupational histories were relatively well-defined in the Case study because of the availability of employer records. The control population, as well as the exposed population, had appropriate adjustment to clarify and standardize secular variations in diagnoses as well as exposure. The nature of the disease is such that end results should lead to relatively few case losses. Since only cases on the nominal employer rolls were utilized by Case, biases arising out of the tendency to add cases later found in hospitals or other death-certificated cases was minimized. This course of action would tend to underestimate the risk thus making even more impressive the degree of hazard found.

In view of the problems in experimental reproduction of the tumor, there has been a reluctance on the part of some to consider the evidence thus far adduced as conclusive. Considering the history of similar difficulties inducing experimental cancers with BNA, such reluctance places a heavy burden of responsibility on those who minimize the carcinogenicity of benzidine.

Questions have been raised regarding the carcinogenicity of the several salts of benzidine or its precursors. As to the latter, although Barsotti and Vigliani (1949) found no evidence of carcinogenicity among workers exposed only to hydrazobenzine, Scott and Williams (1957) believe this compound can be converted to benzidine upon contact with gastric acids. While benzidine salts, because of their lower vapor pressure, are not a source of vapor contamination, nevertheless they still present hazards because of the possibility of skin and dust exposure.

Chromium

EPIDEMIOLOGICAL EVIDENCE. The study of Bidstrup and Case (1956) indicated, upon the basis of a retrospective cohort study, that the risk of dying from pulmonary cancer in this industry was 360 percent higher than for the general population. Mancuso (1951) examined the records of all employees in a chromate-producing plant, and compared their mortailty experience with all non-chromate worker deaths in the same geographical area. Of 33 chromate workers who were employed for more than one year and who died between 1931 and 1949, 6 or 18.2 percent suffered from lung cancers.

Other studies do not meet the criteria noted previously. The study of Machle and Gregorius was subject to the limitation of small numbers making age adjustment difficult. Diagnoses were not uniformly based upon pathological results while workers who left chromate exposure before their disease developed were not included. Baetjer attempted to remedy these problems, but that study utilizes a control population drawn from hospitals, which could introduce some bias. The study of Brinton *et al.* suffered from shortcomings similar to that of Machle and Gregorius, i.e. the observed number of carcinoma deaths in these categories is probably underestimated.

EXPERIMENTAL EVIDENCE. Until recently it would appear that experimental reproduction of the bronchiogenic carcinoma seen in man has been questionable. However, Laskin *et al.* have succeeded in producing lung tumors with endotrachial calcium chromate; in addition they saw two hepatocellular carcinomata using chromic trioxide. Comparison studies against methyl-cholanthrene (MC) and benzo-a-pyrene (BaP) indicated that while median cancer-time appearances were similar for all compounds, the cancer incidence for calcium chromate and processed residue was considerably less than that of the other two well-known carcinogens, MC and BaP:

Material	*Cancer Incidence*
MC	29.7%
BaP	17.0%
Calcium chromate	6.4%
Processed residue	1.1%
(adapted from Laskin *et al.*)	

This report stands in contrast to numerous previous attempts at bronchiogenic carcinoma induction by various chromates; these produced either sarcoma (by subcutaneous implantation) or at best lung carcinomata by intrapleural implantation (Hueper, 1958). However, Heuper *et al.* repeated such experiments in 1964 and were unable to reproduce their previous lung carcinomata.

USES AND OCCURRENCE. This metal is highly useful material for alloying the nickel, molybdenum, etc. to produce high-temperature corrosion-resistant alloys. It is even more widely used in plating operations, usually in the form of chromic acid. It is also a constituent of corrosion-inhibiting paints and in common use as a tanning agent (hexavalent sodium dichromate), and as a pigment in paints and other coloring agents (in soluble salts as lead and barium chromate and trivalent chromium oxide). It is extensively utilized in the preparation of a large number of chromate compounds.

COMMENTS. Until the Laskin *et al.* report, the hazard to man appeared to be circumscribed to chromate-ore reduction plants, especially in dealing with residues of chromate leaching operations.

It would now seem that more consideration must be given to more than extensive dust and vapor control at numerous points in the chromate reduction process.

Nickel

EPIDEMIOLOGICAL EVIDENCE. The evidence for occupational carcinogenicity rests largely upon the study by Doll (1958) of workers engaged in the manufacture of metallic nickel by the Mond process. Since that process utilizes nickel carbonyl, and because there are no other epidemiological studies available regarding nickel many have been tempted to ascribe carcinogenesis to that particular compound. This is open to serious question, however, since cases (see below) have been reported from a nickel refinery which purified the metal by another process. The suggestion of Morgan that these Mond process cases were due to dusts contaminated with arsenic which were found in that plant is also dubious, since there is no basis at present for implicating arsenic as a causative agent of nasal sinus cancers seen in that exposed population.

The retrospective study of Doll utilized proportional mortality rates and depended upon death certificates collected in the area. No access to plant rolls was indicated. While some secular corrections were applied, little other age correction could be made with the data at hand. Occupational diagnosis depended upon follow-up death certificates by interviewers. While this study suffers from many of the shortcomings of retrospective mortality studies discussed above, the difference in the risk of developing lung tumors (five-fold) and nasal cancers (one hundred and fifty-fold) is so high as to minimize these shortcomings.

EXPERIMENTAL EVIDENCE. Induction of mixed tumors in rats following nickel carbonyl exposure has been reported by Sundermann *et al.* One experiment consisted of a single 1 mg dose (LD50) given to one group of rats; this was reduced by $\frac{1}{4}$ and $\frac{1}{8}$ in another series and was administered chronically. In those animals surviving more than one year (28/176), four tumors were found. The incidence was relatively low.

Hueper (1958b) reported the induction of benign and mixed malignant pulmonary tumors in guinea pigs. He also produced adenomatoid proliferations in rats following chronic inhalation of powdered nickel; Hueper could not produce changes in mice. It should be noted that the dose necessary to produce these responses were quite high, i.e. 15 mg/m3.

CASE REPORTS. As regards nickel, there are relatively large numbers of case reports or collections of cases (Amor, Jones-Williams; Morgan and Løkin), which are largely (except for the last author) associated with Mond process operators.

USES AND OCCURRENCE. This metal is ubiquitous in industry, being mainly used as an alloy with copper, manganese, zinc, chromium, iron, molybdenum, etc. Large quantities are used in plating operations, in metallic anodes and as salts. It is also involved in the hydrogenation of oils, and finds increasing use as an alloy with cadmium in battery manufacture.

Epidemiologic Evidence only

Arsenic

EPIDEMIOLOGICAL EVIDENCE. Until recently strong indicators, but questionably definitive answers—were available regarding arsenic-induced cancer among working populations. While the Hill and Faning study clearly indicated that skin cancers resulted from sodium arsenite exposure, the same report could not draw as definitive a conclusion regarding lung tumors. The reports of Roth, Braun and Osburn depended heavily upon clinical considerations and rough proportional mortality rates, but lacked sufficient population bases to meet more vigorous epidemiological criteria. The matter was further complicated by the reports of Pinto and Bennett, as well as Snegireff and Lombard, which indicated no undue risk of lung cancer.

Recently, however, Lee and Fraumani reported a study involving a working population engaged in metal smelting who had an associated risk of exposure to arsenic trioxide and sulphur dioxide. Few individuals were lost from rolls provided by these smelters, and adequate population bases were constructed; death-certificated diagnoses were the only bases for defining cause of death. These authors concluded that workers exposed to arsenic trioxide incurred risks of lung cancer in proportion to the degree of exposure, such risk being threefold greater than for the general population of that region. While smoking histories were not available, recalculation of their data showed that these workers were at two to two and one-half times greater risks than even heavy smokers. The concurrent SO_2 exposure appeared to enhance the risk; however, it should be pointed out that workers were in the main exposed to both chemicals so that individual effects could not be separated by this study. However, there has not been any suggestion heretofore that SO_2 per se is carcinogenic; its role in impairing respiratory clearance should serve to enhance the carcinogenic process by prolonging bronchial mucosal exposure to an active tumourogenic agent.

The question of ionizing radiation as a contaminant of these ores was considered; the evidence in this regard would minimize such contamination in contrast to the situation among the Schneeberg miners.

It would appear that the evidence for carcinogenicity of arsenic trioxide in the lungs may be as strong as that for sodium arsenite on the skin. Whether these are the only carcinogenic arsenic compounds, however, and whether they are strong carcinogens—e.g. as compared with the aromatic amines—is questionable. Also unanswered at this time is the question of the breadth of the spectrum of arsenic compounds which are carcinogenic. This question must be faced, since arsenic is widely distributed in foods and soils (Monnier-Williams) and is normally found in various body media.

EXPERIMENTAL EVIDENCE. The induction of cancer using arsenic has not been conclusively achieved in any species. Leitch and Kennaway could only produce one metastasising squamous cell epithelioma in one hundred mice with cutaneous application; it should be noted that most of the mice died because of the high toxicity of the dose administered. As regards the general principle of foetal sensitivity to the blastomatogenic action of carcinogens, Askanazy succeeded in developing teratomatous neoplasms in arsenic-treated rat embryos.

USES AND OCCURRENCE. The trioxide AS_2O_3 is commonly found as a contaminant of numerous metal-refining processes (silver, gold, copper, zinc). It is used for the manufacture of economic poisons (such as sodium arsenite), as well as in the glass industry as a decolorizing agent or in production of opal glass. Whereas small amounts may be used in metal alloying, the former large use of arsenic by the pharmaceutical industry has been essentially discontinued.

Mustard Gas — (see Biological Alkylating Agents, page 52).

Group II—Probably carcinogenic
Epidemiologically associated with carcinogens and problematic experimental evidence

4-nitro-biphenyl

EPIDEMIOLOGICAL EVIDENCE. There is no direct epidemiological evidence for the carcinogenicity of this compound. However, in the manufacture of 4-aminobiphenyl, an associated contaminant was 4-nitrobiphenyl. Since the study of Melick *et al.* posed the possibility of exposure to this compound in the course of manufacture of the 4-amino product, and because the 4-nitro compound appears to be carcinogenic to animals (see below), this material is mentioned within that epidemiological context.

EXPERIMENTAL EVIDENCE. Deichmann *et al.* (1958b) reported on induction of bladder cancers by this compound in dogs. It should be pointed out that massive doses were required to produce this result.

OCCURRENCE. As a contaminant in the synthesis of 4-amino-biphenyl.

COMMENTS. While this material cannot be directly indicated as a human carcinogen, in view of its action in dogs, it should be considered as highly suspect. Its potency as a carcinogen is open to some question in view of the doses used to induce these tumors. The possibility of a reduced potency for this nitro compound parallels a similar decrease of carcinogenicity seen upon substitution of a nitro group for an amino group in 2-aminofluorene (Morris *et al*).

Alpha-naphthylamine (ANA)

EPIDEMINOLOGICAL EVIDENCE. The 1954 report of Case *et al.* of the dyestuffs industry included a group of workers believed to have contact with ANA alone; they appeared to have a clearly enhanced risk of developing bladder tumors. The fact that a relatively longer latent period was involved implies superficially that those isomers were less potent. However, Case, correcting for this factor—which may tend apparently to diminish the potency of ANA—suggests that the latter's carcinogenicity is still not negligible, although probably weaker than that of BNA and benzidine.

EXPERIMENTAL EVIDENCE. This compound appears to be at best a weak inducer of bladder tumors in animals (Clayson *et al*, 1958). However, later Clayson and Ashton (1963) could not induce tumors in mice following treatment or 0.01% ANA chloride (freed from BNA by multiple fractional recrystalization) in drinking water.

USES AND OCCURRENCE. (see BNA). Manufacture of alpha-naphthol; widely used in the colour industry for manufacture of sulphonated naphthylamines (naphthionic acid, sodium naphthionate).

COMMENTS. The question of the inherent carcinogenicity of this compound is confusing, since much of the commercial-grade compound contains varying amounts of the beta isomer. Its manufacture by the nitration of napthalene results in the formation of 4 to 10 percent of the beta isomer as a contaminant. While a large number of cases of bladder tumors allegedly caused by exposures to the commercial-grade alpha isomer have been recorded (see 80 cases tabulated by Scott, 86 by Temkin), the question of the role of contamination by BNA is still not clearly resolved by such series. While the same consideration of BNA might be applied to Case's 1953 epidemiological study, the weight of evidence is such that commercial-grade ANA containing 4 to 10 percent BNA could be considered hazardous. A personal communication indicates carcinogenicity however among workers handling BNA-free (less than 1%) ANA.

Experimental evidence and case reports

Beryllium

EPIDEMIOLOGICAL EVIDENCE. No definitive study available.

EXPERIMENTAL EVIDENCE. Malignant lung tumors, in addition to adenomata, have resulted from administration of beryllium sulphate aerosol among 50 percent of 76 rats (Schepers, 1957). This work was corroborated by the production of adenocarcinomas in monkeys exposed to a considerably lower concentration of the inhaled oxide and sulphate by Vorwald and co-workers. Metastasising tumors of bone (sarcomata) have been induced by intravenous injection of beryllium zinc silicate and the silicate alone (Barnes *et al.*, 1950), as well as by inhalation of pure baryllium oxide (Dutra *et al.*).

CASE REPORTS. In his study, Mancuso (1970) attempted to substantiate previous statements by the epidemiological analysis of social security records. He tried to define relative degree of exposure on the basis of work duration, since occupational histories could not be utilized—and were not available. The author assumed equal risk for each reported quarter of yearly employment according to the records; because the number of lung cancer deaths was small that report did not attempt to establish a control population base for comparison. The author did not compare mortality for the relative population of the short-term and longer-term employees; this problem is especially important in view of the apparently higher risk of developing lung malignancies in this large short-term employment group. Whether this population loss was due to normal turnover or solely to the fact that acute disease removed such workers is not clarified.

Although Mancuso's approach could be promising, apparently a longer period of time must be allowed to elapse so that a larger number of deaths can be uncovered.

Sporadic cases of pulmonary and other malignancies have been reported among the workers having had beryllium exposure or beryllium disease (Tepper *et al;* Lieben), but no indication of the frequency of these occurrences is presently available.

USES AND OCCURRENCE. Beryllium alloys with copper, aluminum, nickel Electrodes, X-ray diffraction tubes, fuel element cladding for nuclear reactors.

COMMENTS. While the experimental evidence appears reasonably sound, the question of human cancer potential is open to question upon the application of rigorous criteria of proof. It may be that beryllium is a low-potency carcinogen in the forms which have been associated with human exposure. Thus a long latent period may be delaying the appearance of cases. However, this view is open to question since the manufacture and use of beryllium metals dates back to the early 1930s. Mancuso suggested that lung cancers occurred with a higher frequency among workers who had sustained a previous episode of acute respiratory berylliosis. If individual host factors determine whether such an acute response will occur, self-selection should operate to decrease any subsequent number of cancers, since relatively fewer workers would sustain such acute episodes or would be retained following them. The alternative possibility might be considered, that there is a threshold not only for acute berylliosis but also for development of subsequent cancers. Either circumstances might explain why few tumors have been reported in man.

Case reports only

Benzene

EPIDEMIOLOGICAL EVIDENCE. There is no valid epidemiological evidence incriminating benzene as a leukaemogenic agent.

EXPERIMENTAL EVIDENCE. It is generally accepted that leukemia has not been reproduced in experimental animals, despite the study of Lignac, which is unconvincing.

CASE REPORTS. Despite the absence of adequate epidemiological or animal models, the literature contains many reports of the occurrence of leukemic alteration of the blood-forming elements following benzene exposure. Vigliani and Saita (1964) collected six cases occurring over a two-year period and as recently as 1970. Girard *et al*, surveying 401 hospital admissions for severe haematologic disorders, found twenty-six cases of leukemia allegedly associated with benzene. Social security statistics from the Paris area regarding forty-five haemopathic deaths during the period 1947 to 1961 revealed twenty-one leukemias among benezene-exposed workers (Cavigneaux *et al.*), while in the same region fifty cases were recorded for the period 1950-65 (Goguel *et al.*).

USES AND OCCURRENCE. Synthesis of organic compounds; solvents for organics; as a rubber solvent; used in *sizing* fibres; in paint and varnish; mirror manufacture; artificial leather manufacture.

COMMENTS. While there are extensive case reports and collections of cases in the medical literature concerning the leukemic consequences of benzene exposure, there is at present no adequately constructed epidemiological study of this question. Furthermore, regarding the reproduction in animals of these alleged consequences of benzene exposure, there is at present no adequately constructed experimental study of this question. Thus, the reproduction in animals of these alleged consequences of benzene exposure provides another element of doubt. While the literature suggests that this effect may be the consequences of *special susceptibility*, especially in women, there is no firm basis for this observation.

That most individuals with chronic benezene poisoning *do not* develop leukemia does suggest a special *atypical* type response, similar to the idiosyncratic aplastic anaemias occasionally seen after administration of common therapeutic drugs. Further, the relatively few cases of benzene-induced leukemia have occurred in persons sustaining sufficiently severe exposures to have suffered the usual type of chemical intoxication; yet the vast majority of severe poisonings do not develop leukemia.

Group III—Presumably carcinogenic
Experimental evidence only

Nitrosoamines (N-nitrosodimethylamine, DMN)

EPIDEMIOLOGY. No epidemiological studies of this class of compounds are known.

EXPERIMENTAL EVIDENCE. This compound has been extensively studied in animals, and is a potent carcinogen in at least six different species (mouse, rat, hamster, guinea pig, rabbit and rainbow trout). Neoplasia can be induced through various routes of administration (oral, subcutaneous, intraperitoneal); organ sites vary according to routes of administration or species utilized. In the rat, the malignant tumors were most commonly observed in the liver (Magee and Barnes, 1956) when this material was given in low doses for a longer period of time, or in the kidney (Magee and Barnes, 1962) when given as a single high dose. In addition, in other experiments a relatively high single dose in the mouse produced lung adenomata (Den Englse *et al.*, 1970).

CASE REPORTS. There have been no malignant responses seen among individuals acutely exposed to DMN, although liver damage has been reported in four cases (Freund; Barnes and Magee).

USES AND OCCURRENCE. This material has been used as an industrial solvent and in the synthesis of unsymmetrical dimethylhydrazine, a rocket fuel.

COMMENTS. The extent of industrial use and human exposure is not known. The toxic liver damage seen in humans has also been very frequently encountered in animals. Because of its consistent and potent carcinogenicity in animals, this substance is most probably carcinogenic in man.

Diamino-diphenyls

In this group are 4, 4'-Methylene bio-o-chloroaniline (DACPM) and 4, 4'-Diaminodephenyl-methane (DADPM). Structurally, these consist basically of two benzene rings linked by a methyl group, with animo substituents in the paraposition. In the case of the former, there are single chlorine atoms substituted at 3,3' positions; the latter lacks such chlorine atoms.

EPIDEMIOLOGY. There are no such adequately described human studies.

EXPERIMENTAL EVIDENCE. Twenty-seven grams/kg DACPM given to 50 rats maintained on a low protein diet produced hepatomas and lung tumors in 43 animals (Grundmann and Stcinhoff). These same authors produced hepatomas and 7 primary lung tumors in 34 rats following subcutaneous injection. DADPM, although closely related structurally, appears less carcinogenic than DACPM. The evidence is relatively more equivocal, since in two small series totalling 51 rats a relatively level yield of tumors (10) was found (Schoental, 1968).

USES AND OCCURRENCE. Both are used as curing agents in polyurethane elastomer resins. DACPM is recommended for use in less than stochiometic quantities so that little is probably present as the unreacted chemical. DADPM is converted immediately into a mixture of di, tri and polyamines for production of such foam and elastomers. Less of both agents is also probably used as curing agents for epoxy and epoxy-urethane resins.

COMMENTS. Worker exposure to these agents is likely to occur, especially in small plants and workshops. While the first of these two agents (DACPM) is clearly more carcinogenic than DADPM, their resemblence to other compounds of this class of diphenyls known to produce cancers in humans suggests a serious possibility of carcinogenic risk. In the case of DADPM, its contamination of flour has led to cases of jaundice in 84 persons; however, no cancers have yet been seen among those persons affected (Kopellman *et al.*, 1966).

Biological alkylating agents (nitrogen mustards, imines, epoxides, lactones)

EPIDEMIOLOGICAL EVIDENCE. A retrospective study of Japanese workers manufacturing mustard gas has clearly indicated a marked excess of lung tumors (Wada *et al.*).

EXPERIMENTAL EVIDENCE. Variants of the aliphatic and aromatic nitrogen mustards have consistently given positive results when studied for carcinogenic action. Tumors have resulted locally (as sarcomata) in addition to occurring in distant organs. Specific epoxides have also produced carcinomas and sarcomas (e.g. vinyl cyclohexenediepoxide), as have certain imines (e.g. ethyleneimine). Similar activity has been found for certain lactones (notably beta-propriolactone). Most of the above have not been implicated in human disease except as noted above.

USES AND OCCURRENCE. Several of these poly-functional compounds have been used in industry to modify the characteristics of textile fibers.

Dichlorobenzidine (DCB)
Orthotolidine (OT)
Dianisidine (DA)

EPIDEMIOLOGICAL EVIDENCE. None.

EXPERIMENTAL EVIDENCE. Pliss (1959) produced local tumors after injection with DCB in 75 percent of white mice surviving this study. Seven animals affected showed local sarcomata; two given DCB orally had adenosarcomata of the gastro-intestinal tract. Distant tumors of the liver were reported in twelve rats, while three bladder papillomata were also found. In addition numerous animals were reported as demonstrating mammary and sebaceous gland tumors. This work could not be confirmed by Sciarini and Meigs (1961).

Pliss later (1965) reported that o-tolidine given subcutaneously also produce distant tumors of the sebaceous and mammary glands but no local neoplasia at the point of injection. Scott (1962) reports—via a personal communication from Walpole and Williams—that this compound appeared to be a weak carcinogen. Troll and Nelson (1958) fed o-toldine to dogs for an unspecified period and failed to note the occurrence of tumors. It should be pointed out that their study was directed towards delineation of metabolic pathways rather than carcinogenicity per se. Pliss also reported in his report of 1965 that dianisidine was found to be only very slightly carcinogenic, with tumors developing following oral administration in four of forty-two animals. Once more, Scott reports via personal communication from Walpole and Williams that this compound produced distant tumors. More recently Pliss and Zabezhinsky (1970) induced 101 tumors in 48 of 108 surviving treated rats with purified o-tolidine. Following subcutaneous injection and implantation, Zymbal's gland tumors and neoplasia at other sites were seen.

CASE REPORTS. None.

USES AND OCCURRENCE. Curing agents, pre-polymerization; *azo* dyestuffs; preparation of ion exchange resins.

COMMENTS. All of these chemicals have been closely associated with the manufacture of benzidine. While this might warrant placing these compounds in Group II - Probably Carcinogenic, the available experimental evidence is too weak for such action. However, they are placed in the Presumably Carcinogenic group because their close industrial association with a known carcinogen makes a *sorting out* of the evidence difficult. Accordingly, Scott (1962) recommends that they should be treated in a similar fashion to benzidine in industrial usage.

UNCHARACTERIZED OR CONTAMINATED MIXTURE
Definition

Such materials may exist in complex mixtures which makes difficult their analytical isolation and characterization of specific carcinogenic components. These groups of carinogens may also be associated with other, clearly active, carcinogenic agents, either in their natural or technical forms. In such circumstanes, the relative carcinogenicity of each component may be undetermined or unclear at this time.

Group I - Definitely carcinogenic
Epidemiological and experimental evidence

Mineral-derived oils, coal tars and pitches, etc.

EPIDEMIOLOGICAL EVIDENCE. Faced with a heterogeneous group of materials, it becomes impossible to cite any one study to incriminate the entire group. Accordingly since a number of materials have a common feature, i.e. derivation from mineral sources, any attempts rigorously to review the epidemiological evidence must rely upon some prototypal characterization of these materials.

TARS AND OTHER MATERIALS ASSOCIATED WITH CARBONIZATION OF COAL. Doll's 1965 report was a prospective study which meets the criteria for a well-executed, definitive epidemiological investigation. Appropriate population bases of comparisons were obtained, occupational histories were available from employer rolls, appropriate characterizations and groupings by age were achieved, and the loss of subjects to the study was extremely low. The diagnoses were not histologic, being based upon death certificates; however, the same biases as regards diagnoses should have been operative among control subjects as among study groups.

This report showed a clearly increased risk of lung cancer among those exposed to fumes and gases produced by the carbonization of coal in retort houses. A similar well-constructed cohort study of Kawai *et al.* (1967) arrives at much the same conclusion as the Doll report. In the Kawai study diagnoses were all confirmed clinically or histologically, although all individuals surviving beyond the age of 55 were lost to the study.

Of further interest in the Doll report is the suggestive finding of a strong indication of an increased risk of bladder tumors. This has been noted in other studies (e.g. Bruusgaard). Similar studies, although not necessarily as complete—e.g. in Canada (Sutherland), Norway (Bruusgaard) and Japan (Kuroda)—would appear to confirm the existence of an increased risk of lung tumors among producer-gas workers.

The recent well-constructed retrospective series of studies by Lloyd (1969, 1970 and 1971) previously cited, also meets stringent requirements for adequacy as regards epidemiology. That study clearly indicated a ten-fold increase in the risk of lung cancers among coke-oven workers working on the top of such equipment (cf. Doll, 1965, horizontal versus vertical gas retorts). Suggestions as to excess bladder tumor deaths and carcinoma of the pancreas (cf. Mancuso, 1969) were presented, but the evidence was inadequate clearly to define the risk (cf. Doll, 1965; Henry *et al.*, 1931). It should be noted that beta-naphthylamine has been detected in off-gases of gas retorts (Battye).

MINERAL WAX AND OILS, COAL TAR AND PITCH. A prospective study (Hendricks *et al.*) of the incidence of cancers among mineral oil pressmen indicated a risk of incurring neoplastic disease about four times greater than for the general male population. The fact that the majority of these were scrotal cancers, a form that is allegedly rare, if not nonexistent except with occupational exposure, makes their estimation of total cancer risk rather conservative, since they included scrotal cancer (which accounted for 60 percent of the observed cancers) in the total cancer rate among the exposed group. The ocupational histories were complete, being available from company rolls for those working one day or longer; medical histories as well as tissue diagnoses were also available. Appropriate adjustments for age and occupation were made, as were adjustments for secular variation in the population base. The adequacy of this study of such exposure to petroleum waxes leaves the correlation with scrotal cancer open to little doubt.

Henry's researches were based upon extensive collections of death certificates on a national basis. Despite their extensiveness, these were limited in their ability to meet the epidemiological criteria noted. The problem of attribution of occupation to cases— particularly as reported by both certificates—made the derived data, at best, only approximations. Much the same comment applies to his studies regarding tars and pitches.

EXPERIMENTAL EVIDENCE. Much of the testing of crude products encountered in industry is reported in the literature prior to the first half of the twentieth century. Thus the early reports of induction of skin tumors, e.g. the studies of Passey using extracted soot, the studies of Leitch with oils, or the extensive investigations of Twort, all contribute toward the establisment of bases for a half-century of clinical observations. In addition, because of the extreme degree of constituent variability, this group of crude materials yielded unpredictable results as regards carcinogenesis. Later studies, (e.g. Smith *et al.*), which recognized some of these interacting variables, reproduced skin tumors in several species exposed to various catalytically-cracked petroleum distillates. However, most of these studies were reported prior to the development of an understanding of the interactions of co-carcinogens, promoters or solvents, and of a clearer appreciation of the influence of dose and schedules of administration (see above).

It became clear that several specific compounds which were consistently carcinogenic (e.g. BaP, DBA) were regular components of these materials so that more recently, much investigational activity has been directed towards the testing of these compounds rather than of crude mixtures.

OCCURRENCE. It should be carefully noted that the carcinogenic potency of the mineral-derived tars, pitches and oils is highly variable, depending upon source, method of preparation and distillation, and contents. While the list of exposures may be extensive, it cannot be assumed that the risk of cancer is uniform—or indeed even existent—in all times or places, since the component materials involved in these exposures are highly variable.

The list includes:

Cotton mule spinners	Asphalt industry
Petroleum wax pressmen	Cable preservation
Patent fuel manufacture	Road repairing
Tar distillation	Metalworking
Coke ovens	Still cleaning in oil
Gas workers	refineries

COMMENTS. As noted previously, active carcinogens have been isolated from mineral wax, oils, pitches and tars. However, while such specific compounds have been quantitatively isolated, it cannot at this time be assumed that they are the only carcinogens in such mixtures.

Asbestos

EPIDEMIOLOGICAL EVIDENCE. The early investigations of Merewether reported that the association between asbestosis and lung cancer was significantly more pronounced than between silicosis and that malignancy. These studies may be faulted, since he attempted to set a rate in this relatively uncommon condition for cancer among only 344 individuals with asbestosis. In addition the fact that the designation of *asbestosis* or of *abestos worker* had necessarily to be present on the death certificate before coming to the investigators' attention also probably led to underestimation. The latter criticism was essentially avoided by the study by Doll (1955) or an asbestos plant; while, again, he used coroner's records, each dianogsis was based upon pathological evidence. Indeed, his approach, which only considered workers engaged at the plant for 20 years or more, may have once more underestimated the risk. The population base was the Registrar General's rate for England and Wales, which he then conservatively corrected for the geographic area. The excess lung cancer mortality was striking among these workers; this risk would tend largely to overcome the objection that neither a large population nor a documentation of specific job-associated risk was available. Subsequent multiple studies have shown this association to be so constant that the question of the carcinogenicity of asbestos, following exposure to certain of its forms, appears to be substantially settled.

In addition to carcinoma of the lung, mesothelioma has also been associated with asbestos exposure. This condition is so unusual that questions have been raised regarding its existence; furthermore, the diagnostic criteria are difficult or require complete autopsy. Both the foregoing considerations have led to evident difficulties in retrospective studies. It is this very rarity alone which makes this association between asbestos and mesotheliuma stand out.

Retrospective studies by Selikoff *et al.* and Wagner again point to a constant association of this rare condition with asbestos exposure. Although these studies suffer from problems common to other retrospective studies, because of the rarity of pulmonary mesothelioma per se and the relative infrequency of intensive asbestos exposure, one would place more credence upon such studies—with due consideration of their associated problems—than would ordinarily be warranted (cf. retrospective epidemiologic study problems).

EXPERIMENTAL EVIDENCE. Lung cancers (largely adenocarcinoma and several squamous cell tumors) were successfully induced in rats by inhalation exposure to chrysotile (Gross *et al.*). While this cancer was not seen in about 10,000 rats previously examined by the authors (strain unspecified), their ability to induce such tumors in animals stands in contrast to the apparent inability of other investigators (e.g. Wagner *et al.*) using the inhalation technique.

Occurrence and exposure.
Fireproof fabrics
Insulation
Brake linings
Roofing shingles
Clutch plates
Filter cloths

COMMENTS. The assignment of carcinogenicity to asbestos appears clear; what remains clouded is an understanding of which form, fiber, sizes and/or co-factors appear to be responsible for a wide variability in response. There are severe differences between investigators regarding which mineral type, source, fiber characteristic, contaminant, etc. is responsible for neoplastic change. The role of cigarette smoking as an important co-carcinogen has been emphasized by Selikoff (1968). Futhermore, there are suggestions (experimental, case reports) that carcinogenesis involving other mesothelial surfaces may be induced.

Accordingly, while such reservations are specifically directed towards resolving these more specific questions, it would be well to consider this material per se as being under a severe indictment of carcinogenesis.

Epidemiological evidence only

Haematite

EPIDEMIOLOGY. The studies of Boyd *et al* utilized the proportional mortality method, and comparisons were made between the occurrence of death-certificated cases of lung cancer, all other cancers and all other causes. Underground haematite miners were compared with surface workers at the same mines; the same causes-of-death breakdowns were established for coalminers in the same area. Finally, the mortality experience for both groups (i.e. haematite and coalminers) was compared with all other deaths in the area. The death certificate study was extended by a search of hospital records; this resulted in more lung cancer deaths being ascribed to haematite workers. In addition, this extension of the investigation led to the discovery of still more deaths in cases where death certificates failed to mention *haematite mining* as the occupation of the decedent. However, despite the discovery of these additional cases, such cases were not included by the investigation in their estimations of mortality. Hence the 75 percent increase over expected mortality in underground haematite miners probably represents a conservative under-estimate.

This study was based upon local, general mortality rates derived from death certificates, utilizing appropriate age adjustments. No cohort analysis could be performed since accurate employment records were unavailable; accordingly this study cannot be considered as providing a direct measurement of risk. There were, however, internal consistencies which tend to strengthen this study.

EXPERIMENTAL EVIDENCE. Saffiotti *et al.* showed that haematite activated the carcinogenic effects of tar droplets instilled intratracheally in hamsters. Earlier, Campbell's 1940 studies indicated that iron oxide, in association with precipitated silica (influences the induction of primary lung tumors in mice. The foregoing are the experiments whose conditions most closely approximate exposures of concern here. However, work with a complex of ferric oxide and dextran produced high yields of subcutaneous sarcomas at injection sites in a significantly high number of mice (Haddow and Horning), although this study is probably not relevant to the haematite question.

CASE REPORTS. Roussel *et al.* reported over 200 cases of lung cancer in haematite miners in Lorraine. The cases were derived from the clinical records of the Lorraine Anti-Cancer Center and were all confirmed histologically. Work histories were obtained solely from hospital records. The estimate of the risk in this occupation was obtained by classifying the number of lung cancers by occupational groups among these hospital records; the ratio between the percentage of haematite miners with cancers in hospital and the percentage of haematite miners in the working population in that region was calculated. There was no age correction, and no breakdown of workers by occupation in the haematite extraction industry was available. The problem of a possible bias because of the Center being a referral center which may draw patients on a self-selecting basis was not investigated. While this is an impressive series of cases, the treatment of the data leaves a number of questions unanswered. Other similar clinical studies have been derived from this area, notably that of Monlibert and Roubille, who compared the frequency of pulmonary malignancies among 10,000 haematite miners and a similar number of metalworkers. These authors found 64 such cases among miners versus 28 in metalworkers. Unfortunately no data are given for the area on the incidence of lung cancer in the general male population.

COMMENTS. There appears to be a strong suggestion of increased risk of lung cancer among haematite miners. The studies cited (and others) find characteristically an increased incidence of undifferentiated or oat-cell type tumors. The question of the aetiological agent is unclear, since in the Cumberland haematite mines the levels of radon range between 30 pCi (Picouries) to above 300 pCi per liter of air. Roussel *et al.* commented that the radiation levels in the *ores* of Lorraine do not appear to be elevated. However, as pointed out by deVilliers and Windish, the radon in the Newfoundland fluor-spar mines is carried in mine water; thus if only ore samples are measured they could quite possibly be misleadingly low. Furthermore, measurements of ore samples removed from the mines may produce a misleading picture, since radon or its short-lived daughters may no longer be residual in such extracted ores; this has been confirmed by the measurements of Duggan *et al.* in the Cumberland haematite mines. In-mine measurements of radioactivity were elevated, in sharp contrast to Faulds and Stewart's 1956 measurements of the ores *removed* from the mines.

The question of the carcinogenicity of relatively pure iron oxide as encountered in the metal trades is thought-provoking. Kennaway and Kennaway (1947) found an excess by death-certificated mortality for lung cancer among foundry workers, smith and metal grinders over a 17-year period in the United Kingdom; the ratio between observed and expected mortality approximated the excess mortality rate found by Boyd *et al.*

Group II - Probably carcinogenic
Epidemiologically associated with other carcinogens
Problematic experiments

Magenta

EPIDEMIOLOGICAL EVIDENCE. In the course of the study by Case *et al.* for the Association of British Manufacturers and the dye industry, it became apparent that some suspicion of bladder cancer risk was attached to the manufacture of auramine and magenta dyes. Accordingly, nominal employment rolls were established identifying 332 men manufacturing or using magenta only, auramine only, or both of these dyes; 1,223 men were noted as dealing with aniline only. None of these latter workers had contact with BNA, its alphaisomer, or benzidine. Comparative composite cohorts were developed for determination of expected death rates. The names of deceased workers on the nominal roll were found and their death certificates retrived. While mention is made of a search for hospital records, no data are given for the number of verified histological diagnoses. It was concluded from a finding of six bladder tumors in 85 exposed workers that there was a significant risk of bladder tumor development.

EXPERIMENTAL EVIDENCE. No evidence available.

CASE REPORTS. Five cases of bladder cancer were reported to Scott from a plant manufacturing magenta from o-toluidine.

COMMENTS. The authors clearly state that they have no basis for indicting magenta per se; rather, some carcinogenic agent may possibly be encountered in this azo dye's manufacture. This compound is accordingly placed under the category of "Uncharacterized or Contaminated Mixtures". Because of the small study population (85 workers) exposed to magenta alone, and the small number of tumors, we are inclined to place this material in Group II, "Probably Carcinogenic". Nevertheless, while the study population was indeed small, the level of significant occurrence of bladder tumors was sufficient to lead the industry to treat manufacture of this dye in a fashion indicative of some hazard of bladder tumor induction.

Auramine

EPIDEMIOLOGICAL EVIDENCE. Case and Pearson (1954) established a nominal work roll comprising 238 workers with exposure to auramine alone. Even though statistical analysis indicated a high level of probable association, it should be noted that this conclusion was based on a total of nine bladder tumors.

EXPERIMENTAL EVIDENCE. Bonzer, Clayson and Jull (1956) found six hepatoma in a group of 30 rats fed auramine. Similar results as regards hepatoma were also obtained by Williams and Bonzer (1962) and Walpole (1963) in mice; the potency of auramine appeared somewhat less in this species.

CASE REPORTS. Muller (1933) reported two cases in men making auramine from di-methyleneaniline.

USES AND OCCURRENCE. See Magenta.

COMMENTS. The study population, while relatively larger than the magenta group, yielded a total of nine cases of bladder tumors. The level of probable association was statistically significant; the small number of cases plus the fact that Case and Pearson could not state that it was auramine per se which was carcinogenic somewhat vitiates the proof of association. Nevertheless, prudence would indicate that manufacture of this material should be considered as carrying some risk of bladder cancer induction and that it should be handled accordingly.

Chapter III

PREVENTION AND CONTROL OF OCCUPATIONAL CARCINOGENESIS

O N SUPERFICIAL CONSIDERATION it might appear more pertinent at this point to consider that carcinogenic potential in and of itself determines control options. However, if it is our aim to prevent risk of occupational cancer, there is sufficient reason to consider that the realities involved in control may in part operate independently of an individual agent's carcinogenic potential per se. This conclusion stems from actualities that place real limits upon the use of certain carcinogens in industry; such limitations reflect mainly a chemical's mode of usage as well as practical possibilities inherent in control techniques. Both these latter can act independently of carcinogenic potentialities which are based purely upon general principles of biological behavior. For example while the evidence—both epidemiological, if not experimental—for the cancer induction activity of specific chrome compounds is quite strong, the reality of chrome processing indicates a possibility for somewhat more effetive hazard control than is the casc, for example, with beta-naphthylamine. Hence, to examine the evidence for the carcinogenicity of individual or groups of compounds independently of control potentialities is to ignore the realities of the industrial scene.

ABOLITION OF CARCINOGENESIS IN TRADE AND ITS IMPLICATIONS

While this approach to control may have been theoretically more feasible twenty years ago, with the explosive growth in the number of compounds incriminated as having carcinogenic properties such a simplistic approach may now become more difficult. Accordingly, if this method of control is to be seriously considered, even if only for a rare compound, the basis and ramifications of such an action require serious consideration.

Consideration governing use of substitutes

It would appear upon first consideration that the problem of an almost never-ending stream of new chemicals carries both a threat, and a promise. The threat represented by their multiplicity has been dilated upon previously; the promise of this plenitude lies in the implied potentiality for finding or developing substitutes. One therefore finds it difficult to believe in the absolute non-existence of substitute materials.

Accordingly, it would appear that questions of practicality of chemical substitutes ultimately revolve about matters of economics viewed in the light of social goals.

Economic ramifications of abolition

Each of the industries wherein carcinogenic substances are known to be manufactured or employed may loom large as producers of goods and investment return. Each therefore provides employment for some number of workers, both directly and indirectly. Each provides some financial base both for the immediate community and for a nation at large. Accordingly abolition can result in the following economic losses:

1) *Loss of capital investment*—Variable in extent, depending upon recovery by amortization or by ability of operation to be modified to produce a substitute or other product. The last essentially may amount to a salvage program with relatively low capital recovery. Such an approach may often require governmental reimbursement or subsidy.

2) *Loss of employment opportunity*—Variable in extent, depending upon the possibility for shifting workers within a multi-product line plant, or of changing product. Where such plants produce a single product or are small in size, unit shutdown will cause immediate income loss, unless social or worker security schemes underwritten by the government or employers are applicable. In areas of labor

surplus, such benefits should provide for long-term protection; otherwise loss of employment in such areas will lead to long-term or permanent employment loss and individual economic handicap. Retraining schemes can alleviate industrial hardship situations, but once more in areas of labor surplus may not provide permanent solutions to individual worker problems.

3) *Loss of production income*—The ramifications of these losses extend from the immediate community through all intermediate levels and finally to the country as a whole, and include possible national disadvantage in international trade position. At the local and regional level, markets can be depressed with the potential for consequent political repercussions. While some national income encroachment can be expected, there could also be an associated national economic loss through diminution of exports following abolition. In importing nations, an unfavourable influence upon the balance of trade may result if a more expensive substitute is required which they cannot produce. This latter possibility could be considerable among emerging nations; they could be placed at a trade disadvantage in the event that a more *expensive* (financially, technologically) substitute eventually appeared.

In actuality, the foregoing represents the extreme cases. It presupposes in many cases absolute shutdown of production facilities and supernumeration of all involved employees. It further presupposes that other approaches to hazard control cannot be effectuated and that the production facilities represent a unique technology inapplicable to other profitable purposes. Further, it is questionable that, given the size of the industry under suspicion of presenting severe carcinogenic risk, we are considering abolition of any significant proportion of any one nation's gross national product or an important trade balance determinant.

Abolition may be brought about either directly—as by national or International Convention—or indirectly. Should the latter occur it would require total adherence; otherwise an unfair competitive advantage would accrue to the non-complying nation. Further, in some cases it might put technologically advanced nations at an advantage since they could more readily produce more sophisticated substitutes, placing emerging countries in a trade dependency position. Indirect abolition could occur as a result of economics, i.e. the cost of production which requires extensive safeguards might make such a material non-competitive and thus induce obsolescence.

In sharp contrast to economic questions stands the matter of social necessity of those specific materials which might be considered candidates for abolition. How many workers are at risk of developing occupational cancer and what is the cost of human wastage balanced against local and national economic needs? The absolute number of workers supernumerated by abolition—in view of the relatively few candidate-products for abolition being small— is probably not large in total. If this is true, the economic loss in the over-all perspective is probably not significant. The loss to society as a whole through abolition is probably not considerable, unless abolition was proposed for a large number of materials; such is an unlikelihood. Such losses as are represented by somewhat less color-fast garments, or less transparent printing inks, do not loom as large as such other actions that might need be considered, e.g. those that might cause significant threats to important social requirements, as in the abolition of the use of pesticides which could lead to diminished food availability.

TECHNICAL (I.E. ENGINEERING) CONTROL OF CARCINOGENIC RISKS TO INDUSTRIAL WORKERS
General Environmental Control via Technical Measures— Premises and Realities

Short of total and absolute containment (if such in reality exists), control is based upon the premise that some Maximum Allowable Concentrations (MAC) can exist for carcinogens, for to assume that some such value does *not exist immediately* leads to a serious constriction of options, i.e. essentially, total abolition of any carcinogenic material in trade or commerce. Accordingly, some consideration of the premises inherent in MACs should be undertaken, to determine whether such premises or principles are applicable to carcinogenic substances.

Implicit in the setting of MAC values is the assumption of a period (14-16 hours per day) on non-exposure, during which time the body burden of an absorbed chemical returns to a normal or pre-exposure level via metabolic or excretory processes. It is also presumed that such processes do not cause decrements in the ability of the involved metabolic systems to function effectively in the future, i.e. such systems restitute to at least a pre-exposure status— or better—without permanent alteration in function.

The biological action of carcinogens leads to some problems concerning the applicability of these premises inherent to the MAC. For one, with the exception of the immune-type response, the reaction between a toxic chemical and a cell is essentially an *all-or-none* phenomenon occurring within a relatively restricted time period; i.e. following some biochemical or structural alteration the cell either survives holistically intact, or it succumbs. By contrast, it appears that tissue contact with a carcinogen allows for a third possibility, i.e. the cell's replicative or homeostatic control mechanisms may be permanently altered—without immediate expression of such change—resulting in possible neoplastic behaviour at some time in the future. Because cellular alteration persists long after the carcinogen is gone from the cell's milieu, each such injury is cumulative; this is in contrast to non-cumulative injury (within the limits of survival of a number of cells sufficient to carry out organ function) which terminates with cell recovery and/or worker removal from exposure. It is also because of this occult process, impossible to detect or characterize and made up of individual cellular *incidents*, that the shape of the lower range of the dose-response curve has been obscured. This in turn has made even more difficult the determination of a *threshold.*

Further complicating the use of MAC values is the reality of our multi-compound environment. Whereas this is a general problem in the use of MAC values, nevertheless this is mitigated for non-carcinogenic chemicals since, in order for some response to occur, a temporal simultaneity of action is usually required. By contrast, such temporal simultaneity of exposure to two different carcinogens is probably not required in view of the persistent damage potential following one exposure. In addition, with the relatively higher thresholds for the majority of toxic chemicals, such additive—or even—synergistic—effects can usually be anticipated, and the appropriate control action can be more readily taken in the work environment. At the same time the probability of contact with other toxicants in the general environment which approach thresholds associated with deleterious effects is relatively low. This is in marked contrast to the synergistic interaction of a wide variety of carcinogens, co-carcinogens or promoters, which can, at quite low doses, raise above a threshold level the effects of contacts with sub-threshold doses (if such exist) for carcinogens. Further, this promotional effect appears non-specific. Because of the relatively low doses at which promoters are effective this widens immensely the range of potential additive, if not synergistic, interactions in contrast to non-carcinogenic chemicals.

Another element considered in developing of MAC values concerns the question of safety margins between threshold levels of effect and a proposed MAC value itself. Implicit in the choice of, for example, a tenfold margin between lowest dose producing the least effect and a MAC value, is the concept that the least serious effect is usually not life-shortening and is, at the most, temporarily irritating. Since the carcinogenic response can be most readily produced by sub-toxic concentrations of such chemials, obviously the use of this procedure for setting carcinogenic MAC values is inappropriate. Hence, in combination with the extensive possibilities for synergistic or cumulative interactions, the problem of setting the MAC values becomes highly complex.

To place these questions in a proper perspective, there is minimal evidence that a *no-effect* level for carcinogens does exist (Cf. Horten and Denman, 1955, 4-MC and 3,4BaP; Druckrey *et al*, 1962, for 4-dimethylaminoazobenzine; Miller and Miller, 1971). Mantel has suggested that since carcinogenic hazard never completely disappears, that a 100 million-fold safety factor might be taken as an arbitrary standard. Implicit in this suggestion is the concept that such margins probably provide safety only by extending the latent period far beyond expected lifespans. Furthermore, it is apparent now that the possibility exists for enzymatic repair of damage to DNA, and that repeated exposures to carcinogens may not be additive if the period between exposures is sufficient to allow *cellular recovery* to occur (Wynder *et al*.).

On balance, it would appear that MAC values as applied to

carcinogens are presently inappropriate. However, it becomes ultimately necessary to consider these questions within a quantitative frame of reference before settling upon such a position. The literature (experimental and epidemiological) contains *suggestive* evidence of a wide spectrum of carcinogenic *potencies* among even a smaller group of chemicals analogues. With a full realization of the problems inherent in scaling relative potency (Cf. Arcos, Argus and Wolf), as long ago as 1939, Iball, rating carcinogenicity of 20 polycyclic hydrocarbons—on the basis of incidence and latent period of induction of epithelial tumours—demonstrated a range between highest and lowest potencies of 2,160 percent. In view of the difficulties of the experimental method, one should also examine this reality of a spectrum of carcinogenicity based upon human experience.

Reviewing the literature on human experience with carcinogenic agents provides a parallelism as regards the variability of potency of carcinogenic agents. While an extremely high proportion of men exposed to beta-naphthylamine eventually develop bladder tumors, such a relatively uniform response does not appear to occur on exposure to benzene or chromates (Case and Bidstrup). Indeed, the difficulty of obtaining—and the low frequency of response with—experimental exposure to chromates (Laskin *et al*, Hueper, 1958) suggests a relationship between experimental data and human experience which reinforces the concept of a variable range of carcinogenic potencies.

It would appear that they may be a mean between the extremes of absolute prohibition of any carcinogen versus application of some of the principles utilized to set MACs for toxic chemicals. Nevertheless, where such position lies that would permit one development of MACs for carcinogens is at present not discerible. Lacking such information, it would not appear feasible to suggest MAC levels for carcinogens at this time.

Total Isolation of Carcinogens in Industrial Processes

While theoretically such procedure might prevent worker exposure to a carcinogen, in actuality practicality provides at best a minimization of exposure. Accepting this viewpoint, one is then faced with consideration of what such an approach involves vis-a-vis production, since the engineering or technical problems of enclosure design and operation are not inconsiderable.

It is self-evident that enclosure means that a complete barrier be placed between an industrial process and the worker. While visual observation of the process can be obtained via view-ports, manipulation must be achieved via man-machine linkages, e.g. remote manipulators, remote reading instruments, etc. This imimmediately imposes economic restraint upon the operation, in addition to placing encumbrances upon manipulation. Such mechanical or electronic linkage requires a high order of reliability if the process is to progress on a steady production basis. The ventilation of such enclosures requires a system of high reliability if production needs are to be met; such systems need to be isolated, essentially self-contained units. For certain processes, e.g. filter presses, mechanical isolation requires engineering modification of an increasingly complex nature. Furthermore, such temporal adjustments required by successive process phases places encumbrances upon the ease of their achievement and hence require more mechanical design modifications.

Another problem revolves about maintenance and waste disposal. While it may theoretically be possible to shield the worker from the carcinogenic material, ultimately maintenance requirements will supervene. Immediately, a new dimension is imposed upon the problem. Entry of the enclosure requires that stringent controls be placed upon maintenance operations. In some processes, e.g. the production of cyanogenic aromatic nitrocompounds, this has been achieved by total enclosure of maintenance workers in impervious suits with independent air supplies. The problems of temperature and humidity control within such suits can be controlled, e.g. by the use of the Vortex cooler. However, this imposes once more a significant cost, and a technological capability (both for fabrication and maintenance) which can increase product-cost, especially in the case of a low production-volume material. In addition, there is the problem of worker acceptibility, since such suits are both cumbersome and impose not-inconsiderable work stress.

Both worker and process enclosure present another set of problems relating to maintenance. In the case of carcinogens of a relatively high potency, external contamination of such suits or loading of collection devices required for atmospheric control within such apparatus must be dealt with. For man enclosures, some means is required for assuring that the worker upon doffing, or that suit maintenance personnel engaged in cleaning of such suits be protected from carcinogen contact. Likewise, cleaning of air filters, bag houses, etc., imposes provision for non-contamination of workers involved, again by enclosure of the process or the worker. Finally, disposal of such waste material must be considered so that the end result of these steps does not end with more widespread in-factory or general environmental contamination. In rare cases the material removed may be of sufficient commercial value to justify recovery and recycling; in most cases such waste materials must in all probability be incinerated or buried. Once more, another set of requirements must be met for protection of workers at the combustion apparatus; furthermore, there must be an assurance that such devices are reliably efficient so as to cause total oxidation of such materials. Finally, maintenance entry for repair and replacement of incinerators must assure that no residuals of such wastes remain to contaminate workers engaged in such processes. Other alternatives for disposal might be considered (to be discarded immediately in the case of waterborne disposal), which again impose another set of conditions which must be met, as in the case of burial.

It should thus be seen that total enclosure and isolation imposes a pyramiding set of requirements, and cost, to production. Where such product is a high-volume, relatively high-profit material, such costs may be considered reasonable.

In addition, other considerations of a quantitative nature impose themselves upon the question of practicality. As implied previously, the quantitative question of relative carcinogenic potency plays a role. That is, the feasibility of control is inversely proportional to the carcinogenic potency of a material. In the case of beta-naphthylamine, this material represents one end of the spectrum, while benzene exists at the other end. Further—and related to this question—the number of stages and the nature of the processes where in the carcinogenic material is present as such will determine the practicality of control devices. As to the former, e.g.

beta-naphytylamine, where a product is carcinogenic at multiple points in the production procession, the problems of contamination prevention becomes difficult to achieve. By contrast, where it appears that the compound is carcinogenic, only at circumscribed stages of prodution, e.g. chromate residues following leaching (U.S. Public Health Service) may it be feasible to institute isolation—or replacement of process. However, in this case two favorable factors appear to be possibly operative, i.e. the material may not be highly carcinogenic (Laskin *et al*. on the basis of animal experimentation) and the product volume is sufficiently large so that economics favor isolation or strict engineering control.

Local Ventilation Control

From the foregoing it can be seen that this approach represents a lesser degree of control on the continuum which has total isolation at its other extreme. All of the problems of cost and interference with production and problems of ultimate disposal apply here to varying degrees. Obviously, the prerequisite for even considering the local ventilation approach is that the material must be quantitatively determined to be of a clearly low carcinogenic potency. On the basis of present knowledge, such a requirement as regards industrial carcinogens can infrequently be met.

Not only does this difficulty exist in the use of local ventilation, similar requirements must be met as regards potencies of intermediates or by-products. While increasingly more stringent requirements for consumer product safety may provide more quantitative answers to carcinogenicity, this will not be the case for intermediates (though this possibility may be mitigated for waste or by-products as a result of environmental pollution control requirements). That such information will not probably be forthcoming stems from the fact that the costs of research determination of chemical character, quantities present, carcinogenicity, etc., are not likely to be encumbered by the private sector in the case of intermediates or wastes which have no commercial value. This improbability is enhanced by the almost infinite numbers and complexity of such materials in industrial processes.

Total Enclosure of the Worker

As has been aluded to previously, rarely have such measures been employed in the chemical industry. By contrast, this approach has been widely utilized in the developoment of nuclear energy. It should be recognized that such ventures were developed and are operated on bases which are independent of market economics. Thus while remote handling, total enclosure of worker or process, and other technical approaches have been eminently successful in the atomic energy industry, restraints upon capital investment of operating costs were not originally applied.

Aside from a pyramiding of requirements and costs with technical and personal protective controls, there is the matter of worker acceptance. Whereas it is a work tradition in the nuclear energy industry, total enclosure presents in most cases an entirely new work requirement for the chemical industry. Acute toxicity—with reversibility—has been seen or heard of by chemical workers, which aids in convincing them of the desirability of such protection; by contrast, the long-term risks that require such measures become somewhat more difficult of conviction. While cancer as a threat would be expected to constitute a sufficient stimulus to the use of personal protective or technical control devices, continued working with such materials without the immediate threat of untoward consequences leads to complacency. Thus introduction of such protection requires both intelligent use of equipment and continued education as to the necessity for its use. This educational process requires some delicacy; it requires sufficient stimulation to encourage careful use of equipment, though not too much *stimulus* as to make work a continuing anxiety-producing experience.

Economic Factors Influencing Use of Engineering Control Measures

Obviously all such approaches, enclosure and isolation, local ventilation, worker enclosure, etc., present some economic costs. Such costs should be recognized as not directly contributing to the quality of the product, i.e. they represent non-productive cost encumbrances. These costs can be approximately divided into capital investment, operating and maintenance and disposal costs.

Concerning the capital investment costs, such are dependent upon several variables, one being whether production equipment is already in existence and requires modification or if production equipment is at the design phase. If control devices are to be *add-on* to existing equipment, such additions are usually more expensive because of the existent machinery's imposition of configuration restraints. Furthermore, such *add-on* equipment usually is less effective since product or air-flows or reaction rates have been originally designed or subsequently operated without taking into consideration control modalities. Finally such additions rarely can be made without shut-down, which again represents non-return on capital investment for varying periods of time.

On the other hand, while a plant is still in the design phase, such equipment—while representing a real addition to over-all cost as a non-productive cost encumbrance—is both less expensive and more effective. The latter follows from an ability to develop congruencies of control with production design. Total over-all air, product or reaction flows can be developed to be consistent with demands imposed by control devices. While this all does indeed add to the total capital investment, the cost is somewhat less and the efficiency greater than in the case of *add-ons*.

Similar capital investments are required for both acquisition of personnel protection devices, safeguarding and disposal equipment. In most cases, since almost complete maintenance worker isolation is required, this represents capital investment. While usually some waste disposal equipment is available, some modifications of equipment in existence; e.g. enhancement of combustion performance, may be required.

The cost-feasibility of such control will be dependent in part upon the extent of the process requiring control equipment. If but one step—or a circumscribed portion of the process—requires such controls, this enhances economic feasibility of control. If a material is carcinogenic throughout or at multiple stages in the production process, this extends the costs (v.s.).

Frequently it becomes apparent that local enclosure or ventilation or worker protection is totally unfeasible with specific equipment, e.g. filter presses. Alternate methods, in addition to meaning new equipment investment, may also be associated with greater inefficiencies, for example, replacement of filter presses by centrifuges for dewatering. Also in such cases, product quality may be adversely affected, requiring the establishment of new processes, steps or devices. In addition to such capital costs, slowing of the production process is equated with increased cost.

In some cases, replacement by more automated, enclosed equipment may make for greater operational efficiencies, e.g. replacement of open-pan driers by fluid bed or spray drying. Whether such efficiencies yield cost-reduction benefits depends upon multiple factors, the major being whether production volumes are sufficiently great as to obtain economic advantage by continuous operation and rapid amortization.

Other less apparent costs in the operational category ensue upon control device institution. If production equipment control adjustments are required periodically, inaccessibility of such machinery—whether with total enclosure or local controls—is impeded. This leads to more protracted periods of *down-time* superimposing a cost burden. Further, maintenance of control devices imposes another dimension upon the usual operating costs.

It might be argued that the increased mechanization associated with remote operation would decrease labor costs. Aside from a dubious advantage gained by such a situation in a high labor-cost country, such savings are generally not realized. Unless production per unit worker-cost increases considerably because of modifications, such cost-recovery does not usually occur. Not only must the product concerned be produced in high volume, it must also have a high profit return. Present realities in the international chemical markets make such large production items only in rare instances a high profit-margin product. For these reasons, recovery of capital investments through mechanization induced by environmental control occurs unusually.

Control of Physical and Chemical State

It is a truism that vapor pressure is usually a function of physical state, i.e. as a chemical progresses through the gaseous to liquid to solid phase the vapor pressure generally decreases. Thus on this basis, if theoretically all carcinogens were handled as solids, proportionally less of the compound would find its way to the atmosphere. Since the energy required to convey solids in a fluidic state is relatively high, and since such systems require sophisticated engineering design (to operate as well as maintain), those systems for carrying solids (as dusts, granules, etc.) have a high degree of leakage, particularly at filling or other transfer stations. Thus the net advantage of handling chemicals as solids tends to disappear. However, combining solids and liquids (though not those with solvent properties) to form slurries alleviates this problem. Removal of the residue of chromate leaching tanks in a moist state in Great Britian was believed to account for Bidstrup's (1951) finding of no unusual incidence of pulmonary carcinogens among chromate ore production workers. (The actual efficacy occurring from handling chromate leaches in the different physical state was however found to be illusory following Bidstrup's follow-up study of 1956.) Furthermore, such slurries, if spilt, eventually dehydrate so that dust or particulate contamination ensues.

Handling materials in a liquid state theoretically obviates dust contamination. If conveyed in totally closed systems this would avoid the volatilization potential. Realistically, all such systems leak at valves, glands or joints and at various other sites dependent upon thermal or corrosive properties. Replacement costs or costs of resistant materials inflate capital and/or operational costs. Finally, maintenance operations must ensue (e.g. valve-seat replacement, packing) with renewed potential for worker and area contamination of some degree. To some extent, this can be prevented, but in the absence of the threat of acute toxic consequences, employee inattention to hygienic detail requires considerable supervisory and educational attention.

Much the same problem applies to handling chemicals in gaseous or vapor form, though to a lesser degree. Yet to a certain extent, chemicals in this physical state are amenable to contamination control. By strict attention to maintenance and equipment operation it would appear that control of carcinogenic risk can be achieved (Doll, 1958) in such a closed gas-bearing system.

Changes in chemical state can alter carcinogenic potential. Thus diazotization or addition to a sulfo group (SO_3H) can minimize the carcinogenicity of bladder tumor inducing aromatic amines. However, there is a risk of the presence of carcinogenic amines in such commercial grade derivatives, e.g. contamination of naphthionic acid with carcinogenic amines. It has been claimed that the carcinogenicity of benzidine is minimized when it is in the salt form, but such chemical change in actuality does not produce a diminished carcinogenicity per se, rather it is only a reflection of a marked decrease in vapor pressure by the consequence of the benzidine being in salt form. Furthermore, production of an altered product, e.g. sulfonated benzidine, requires that such derivatives be chemically stable, sufficiently so as to prevent reversion spontaneously, or because of mishandling. This change in form leads to cost encumbrances, since utilization of this altered compound requires new production machinery for their reconversion.

While approaches which utilize variations in chemical and physical alteration of carcinogens are recommended, these shortcomings should be noted. Further, use of such alterations where possible requires sufficient animal experimentation—recognizing the problems inherent in this approach—to assure the non-carcinogenicity of such derivatives. However, this approach, even where toxicologically indicated, imposes technical impediments to the efficient utilization of such material. In addition, a cost burden is frequently imposed because of the additional equipment and process time necessary to achieve such physical and chemical changes.

The ultimate usefulness of such modifications will be a function of technical ingenuity, legislation or liability stimulation, as well as the commercial value of the material in question. How each of these variables interact will determine whether such approaches might be considered.

MEDICAL CONTROL OF CARCINOGENIC HAZARD
The Pre-placement Examination

A recent limiting factor imposed upon purely medical concerns is legislation—often developed for purely socially desirable reasons—which implies that any selection process is inherently discriminatory. Thus elimination from employment eligibility of women of a childbearing age, or a predilection for older workers may be implied legally to constitute discrimination or prejudice.

While the general desirability of such legislation is indubitable, those responsible for safeguarding the health of the worker should be clearly permitted to fulfill their medical responsibility within the limits of reasonable safeguards.

While predictability of special susceptibility is not usually feasible, such few specific measures to minimize risk as are available should be utilized. Since most occupational cancers are associated with a latent period of 10 to 40 years, it has been suggested that older workers over the age of 40 should be given precedence. However, the risks inherent in this approach of using older workers must be clearly recognized. While *average* latent periods for the carcinogenic amines are 15 to 20 years, reports in the literature indicate the possibility of tumors occurring at shorter intervals after exposure commences. Since no method exists of predicting which worker might run the risk as soon as 10 years after exposure, the shortcomings of using workers 40 years of age are apparent. In addition, given increasingly greater human longevity, or the possibility of a long life span in any one individual, such mortgaging of future life can be seen to be morally dubious.

While the matter of mutagenesis potentials in man is just now becoming clear, because of the known susceptibility of the foetus to certain carcinogens, women in the child-bearing age should be considered in regard to carcinogenic exposures as representing elevated risks.

Personal hygiene of the applicant should be carefully reviewed to reject nail biters or the bearded because of enhanced oral or respiratory absorption risks. Other indicators of inadequate personal hygiene—e.g. diseased teeth, obviously filthy—suggests that habits of personal cleanliness required for hygienic control will probably not be followed. Mouth breathers with nasal obstruction will probably not wear face masks. A sufficient level of worker intelligence is needed in order to ensure their ability to understand the hazard, to participate in training and to exercise self-discipline sufficient to co-operate in necessary hygienic measures. In exposures carrying a risk of lung tumors non-smokers would be the most desirable job applicants; the reality of such a requirement is quite another question. Previous and present health status would counsel rejection of individuals with past or present disease of those organ systems at risk. This does not necessarily follow from any specific predilection for cancer of such organs; rather the pre-existence of disease will confuse delineation of changes subsequent to exposure. Precancerous lesions of any type must not be present. It is also important that careful previous employment history be obtained. Thus those with previous exposure to carcinogens would be ill-advised to extend the duration of exposure. Aside from these specifics, general standard levels of physical fitness apply.

As to the practicality of these measures, aside from the legalistic problem of non-discrimination alluded to above, other realities are imposed. The nature of the available labor market will determine whether age or sex restrictions are practical. The general standard of living will to some extent limit the degree of personal hygiene facilities available to the population. While intelligence is not necessarily a function of educational opportunity, short of psychological testing such determinations are notably subjective. Since smoking or its prohibition is undoubtedly bound up in cultural practices, rejection upon this basis may be less than practical.

It should be apparent from the foregoing that application of medical criteria to selection of workers is, in some part, subjective. Accordingly, this requires that the industrial physician be wholly familiar with the intimate technical details of the work setting and the socio-economic status of the area, while keeping in mind the potential short-term conflict between production requirements and worker protection. It should be apparent that a high degree of medical discretion must be exercised, since only by the application of such professional judgement can these criteria be equitably applied.

Periodical Examination and Medical Monitoring

The relatively poor record—even of the most technologically advanced medical capabilities—to affect cancer mortality rates has one overriding implication: present diagnostic and therapeutic modalities, in men, for the early detection and cure of cancer are discouragingly inadequate. This immediately places an important limit upon the efficacy of medical control or periodic health examinations. The optimum yield from this procedure would require that early, definitive diagnosis be coupled with efficacious therapy. Whether any medical control procedures represent a prophylactic rather than a diagnostic approach is open to question.

A major factor determining the success of medical monitoring is the accessibility of an occupational cancer to observation. Assuming reliable medical surveillance and well performed self-examination, skin cancers yield the highest probability of early detection and cure. For bladder tumors, medical control measures available are open to question as regards successful prevention once the carcinogenic processes have started. As regards the use of cytologic examination of urinary sediments, a wide spectrum of experience indicates a range of opinions from low utility (Al'tganzen, 88 percent false negatives with patients with tumors) to relatively high detection potential (Crabbe *et al.*, 6 percent false negatives). Critical evaluation of this literature indicates that cyto-diagnosis of initial tumors carries the potential for the extremely early diagnosis of such cancers (Poole-Wilson), while results of such tests in established tumors are apparently less reliable. Others have concluded that cyto-diagnosis alone does not prove satisfactory and have advocated routine cystoscopy. Their contention is based upon the possibility of false negatives which exist even in the reports of the most optimistic cyto-diagnosis advocates (e.g. Crabbe *et al.*). Given the discomfort and possible complications of cystoscopy, the acceptability of this procedure to workers is nevertheless hotly contended. In some nations routine prophylactic cystoscopy appears readily accepted. In the Soviet Union (Temkin) and Switzerland (Muller, 1951) it is reported as being freely accepted; in France (Billiard-Duschesne), Italy and USA (Wolfe) such procedure is less readily volunteered, while in the UK (Goldblatt, 1949) and West Germany extreme resistance is encountered. Essentially the choice revolves about a decision as to the level of acceptibility of false negatives taken in light of worker acceptance of the cystoscopic procedure. Certainly, highly trained medical specialists in either case are required, though training of cytologic technicians is more readily feasible in countries with a relative dearth of urologic specialists.

The relative accessibility of bladder tumors to inspection stands in contrast to the essentially occult nature of early occupational tumors of the nasal sinuses and lungs. In the case of the former, first symptoms or signs depend upon the presence of bleeding or roentgenographic shadows which essentially indicate relatively advanced growths. The same situation has been repeatedly reported as regards X-ray diagnosis of lung tumors. While cytodiagnosis using deep cough sputa has been attempted with cancers here, this procedure can lead to an operational dilemma, i.e. early changes of cytology pose the problem of localization required for surgical intervention. The same problem probably awaits us at such time as a sero-diagnostic method for cancer appears.

Another method of medical monitoring for environmental exposure depends upon the determination of the presence of a chemical or its metabolite in biological media. In the atomic energy industry, analysis of gross urinary alpha or beta activity of workers potentially at risk of internal deposition of radionuclides constitutes a useful, rapid assessment of the degree of exposure. In the case of chemical carcinogens, measurement of the element per se, e.g. chromium, nickel, could be useful in monitoring worker exposure. Regarding measurement of metabolites of carcinogenic amines, techniques for their isolation and identification plus the problem of multiple metabolitic products makes bioassay impractical at this time.

However, the usefulness of bioassay is also limited by three major variables:

1) the availability of sufficiently specific and sensitive methodology, applicable in a *mass production* basis;
2) an understanding of the kinetics and character of the human metabolism for the chemical in question;
3) a knowledge of the relationship between concentrations in the workplace and in biological media.

The first problem is rapidly being solved—especially for the metals—as technology utilizing physical modalities approaches the picogram level of sensitivity. Concerning the second problem, our knowledge of the kinetics of human metabolism rests on somewhat less secure grounds, while characterization and understanding of the significance of various metabolites, e.g. of carcinogenic amines, in man is even more tenuous. Finally, even if the foregoing requirements have been met, a body of knowledge must be available which can accurately correlate multiple concentration levels in biological media with multiple levels of environmental exposure. Here our knowledge—with only few exceptions for non-carcinogens—is unfortunately almost non-existent.

The last condition—assuming the first two are met—from a practical viewpoint controls whether bioassay is applicable. Emphasis on this requirement arises from the realization that unless a statistically significant correlation exists between several levels of exposure and body burden, one is unsure of what bioassay is measuring. Indeed, the possibility must be considered that one might be measuring a degree of over-exposure. While such measurements are of some value, their use is limited to their being only a *component* part of a control program consisting of other pre-danger level indicators. As a corroborator of other overexposure such as semi-quantitative measurements, they serve some useful purpose. The danger in their use stems from a complacency that such purported *quantitative* measurement may elicit, particularly in that they may indicate danger after the fact.

In summary, while medical control measures are recommended, their prophylactic limits must be clearly understood. In most cases this is essentially a function of the location of the occupational cancer. Further, given the matter of availability of medical resources, medical control of occupational cancer again becomes only marginally feasible in itself, though it clearly provides some contribution to control in conjunction with other measures.

HYGIENIC CONTROL

PERSONAL PROTECTVIE DEVICES. Such represent less than adequate control approaches compared to engineering measures which do not depend upon worker discipline or co-operation. While occupational carcinogens are usually inhaled or absorbed percutaneously, measures designed to prevent ingestion must also be utilized. Work clothing must be provided. These cannot be permitted to leave a plant; working clothing lockers should be separated in space from where street clothing is kept and such clothing must be changed at least once a week—probably more frequently, depending upon circumstances, e.g. spills. Indeed, daily change is the only possible (though questionably effective) procedure with clothing liable to absorb carcinogens, i.e. the amines. Attention must be given to the laundering process since cleansing might lead to solubilization of carcinogenic compounds. Chemical testing of clothing has been recommended to ascertain the presence of residual carcinogen (Butt and Stafford).

All special protective clothing, such as gloves, aprons, footwear, must be made of such material which is chemically impervious; this may therefore require the use of relatively more expensive material than rubber, e.g. butyl, vinyl polymeric material. Whereas cotton clothing not ordinarily in contact with carcinogens is used, such cheaper material should be tested for its impervious nature before initial use, regardless of supplier claims. Any such clothing which is contaminated on its inner surface may require discarding, depending upon the ability to assure decontamination. Such garments should have their external surfaces thoroughly washed after each shift. Attention to their state or repair should be a clear responsibility of equipment supply and maintenance units. Training in the use of such garments must emphasize proper use and care and requires frequent reinforcement, since such equipment presents an encumbrance to work with which can lead to operator misuse.

Masks or air-supplied hoods must be provided where dusts or vapors are encountered. Such require proper maintenance and cleansing after use. Dust respirators or cotton wool pads are inadequate, the former because of problems of ensuring adequate fit and usage.

Provision of showers, separate locker rooms for street and work-clothing and paid time for bathing before leaving the premises should be mandatory. Similarly, accidental contamination requires immediate clothing removal and careful showering. The use of scrubbing brush and mail cleansing may be required, as well as hair washing. Segregation of eating places must be rigorously enforced.

Despite the use of all of these measures, this approach suffers from considerable inadequacies unless a continuing educational and supervisory program is pursued. In dealing with materials lacking acute or immediate effects, continual attention to such programs is obligatory since under these conditions worker attention to necessary details of usage becomes lax.

Other hygienic measures to control or minimize exposure, such as limitation of hours of work or number of people exposed should be undertaken. Thus *overtime* should not be permitted except in emergencies, clearly defined as non-repetitive, isolated incident. Further, if men work part of a shift, a bath and complete change is required before going on to other work. The number of employees selected to work in such operations should be kept to an absolute minimum as should the use of temporary or casual workers. Indeed, the latter should not be permitted. Cross transfers should be avoided, and selected contingency employees should be designated in the case of absence of regular workers. Access to such areas within the plant should be strictly controlled. Because of possible limitations upon their ability to be upgraded, pay scales should be adjusted so as to provide the same financial opportunities available to other workers for employees limited in their job mobility to processes wherein a carcinogenic risk exists. It should be clearly recognized that this should *not* be construed as hazard pay if effective safeguards in these operations are feasible and existent.

Careful record-keeping covering all persons engaged in these operations as regards exposure to possible carcinogens is required. This need and the difficulties thereto attendant particularly reflects the long latent period between exposure and tumor appearance, as well as the fact that short exposure (several months for beta-naphythylamine) may induce tumors. The problem of follow-up is aggravated since workers long gone from employment rolls may develop tumors without the knowledge of their former employers. Thus co-ordination of the plant physician with local physicians and public health authorities is indicated; the practicality of such measures may be a function of the available degree of official health agency development.

THE ROLE OF EDUCATION IN THE CONTROL OF INDUSTRIAL CARCINOGENIC RISK

The only possible hope of coping with these problems is by continuing to interface knowledge (animal experimentation, epidemiologic) in the field of chemical carcinogenesis with the development of industrial technology. The burden of this charge is upon industries; it would require that they be thoroughly cognizant of all reports regarding *all* compounds with which they actually or potentially work. It should devolve upon them to be alert regarding the compounds which they use, either identical with or generically similar, that may be associated with carcinogenesis. Even if this is possible, this would not guarantee safety, since the absence of data of carcinogenicity among chemical analogs secures nothing.

Another element of education relates to chemists and other technologists. Such education regarding carcinogenic risks should be imposed both during the formal educational process and on a continuing basis during their professional lifetimes. Unfortunately, the present reality is such that chemists—who should know better—are negligent in their handling and usually ignorant or minimizing of the carcinogenic capacity of the chemicals they deal with. Efforts directed towards this matter have not been sufficiently considered or effectuated in the past.

THE FEASIBILITY OF ENGINEERING CONTROL
General Considerations

Given the foregoing appreciation of the limitations attendant upon technical control measures, a balanced overview and conclusions regarding the feasibility of manufacture of carcinogens is useful. The major factors discussed previously when applied to specific compounds will determine the practicality of such manufacture. However, all these factors derive from two major considerations, viz: 1) the inherent carcinogenic potency of the material in question and 2) the extent throughout the course of the process to which the chemical is carcinogenically active. These two questions cannot be considered independently of each other, since a strong indication of intrinsic carcinogenicity may not preclude safe manufacture if the response to the second question suggests a circumscribed risk.

For example, on the basis of its potency, safe manufacture of BNA would appear difficult—but not necessarily impossible—because of the fact that it is highly active throughout multiple stages of synthesis and usage. By contrast, while nickel carbonyl appears to be a potent agent, the fact that it exists in only circumscribed phases of nickel purification (plus, it is a readily confined gas) places this compound in a different category.

Accordingly, if in the light of such considerations it appears feasible to undertake manufacture, an outline of the required technical or engineering control measures where it should be used becomes pertinent.

Building Construction and Ventilation

In order to prevent contamination which cannot be readily removed from surfaces, the use of wood for construction should be obviated. Floors should be designed to permit adequate drainage and should be made of wear and chemical-resistant materials that prevent cracking and subsequent accumulation of spills. Such building should be isolated from other processes and entry must be limited to only those personnel under permanent health supervision.

Forced ventilation of such buildings is mandatory so that combined with a relative negative pressure in equipment, leaks tend to flow *into* apparatus. Because of this need to maintain adequate building air flow, individual air trunks may be required for at least each floor. Ventilation intakes must be carefully located sufficiently far from vent locations. Process vents should be directed away from the building or its neighbors and scrubbers should be utilized. Vents on reactors and other vessels should be so designed so that upon their being filled displaced air is not vented; rather such air vapor mixtures should be conducted back to the storage reservoir which is the source of the material being added.

General Principles of Equipment Design

Wherever possible any manual material handling which involves carcinogens or contaminated mixtures must be eliminated. It is in the plant design phase that the most effective control measures can be applied. All materials used should have a high degree of corrosion resistance to obviate frequent maintenance activity; layout should consider the necessity for simple disassembly and replacement. Pipelines should avoid sharp angles to avoid blockages. Risk of exposure upon handling materials is minimized when they can be moved as liquids, i.e. in slurries or solutions. Ultimately, product transportation costs require conversion of such liquid mixtures to water-free states; it is this step which leads to design and handling problems.

CONTROL OF OPERATIONS. Weighing and sampling material preparatory, during and after synthesis operations present multiple opportunities for worker exposure. Where solids instead of liquids or gases are handled this problem becomes more acute, unless enclosure and ventilation of weighing and sampling stations is accomplished. Automatic sampling and level measuring equipment can minimize the problem, e.g. melting point, pH determination, etc. All manual dipper sampling or dipstick level measurements should be eliminated.

STILL OR REACTOR CLEANING. This requirement may pose difficult hazard control problems. In addition to the economic burdens of equipment *down-time* which ensue when residue sets hard in a vessel, the health hazard involved in such clean-up is severe. The problem of clean-up can be avoided in part if still molten residues are fed directly to an incinerator for complete combustion. While hand-cleaning of reaction vessels may be less expensive than use of solvents, the problem, associated with the use of air supplied suits—with their supporting and cleaning costs—might recommend the latter. Certainly, from the point of view of control, solvent cleaning is preferable.

FILTERING AND DRYING. Ultimately most products require filtering and drying. Enclosure and ventilation of very large rotary kilns has been accomplished where demanded by environmental control reasons. For smaller drying operations methods which minimize man-exposure are available, e.g. filter presses should be replaced by self-emptying centrifuges, rotary or vacuum filters. Tray drying is particularly difficult to control and should be replaced by fluid bed or spray driers where possible. Vacuum stoves present some problem of contamination when first opened. Drum driers can be enclosed though external adjustment of scraper blades may present problems. Grinding of carcinogens should be avoided. When possible, centrifuging to a low water content or spray driying should be substituted.

PACKAGING AND TRANSPORT. These require the use of materials which minimize opportunities for exposure. Here also, transport of solids at packing stations requires highly efficient local ventilation and rigorous use of personal protective devices. Filling should be achieved with use of a relative negative pressure within containers. The use of slurries or liquids leads to more efficient and less hazardous material transfer; accordingly a solid might be remelted (in an exhausted enclosure) before transfer. Heavy guage plastic liners should be inserted into drums to minimize subsequent drum cleaning problems. Adequate instructions for disposal of such liner bags is mandatory; preferably these should be returned by the user to the producer. Remote, exhausted hot water drum cleaners should be used carefully taking care not to discharge their effluents near working areas. Systems should be established for discarding all damaged drums.

MAINTENANCE. This poses many problems previously discussed. Before any equipment is moved from production areas to shops they must be carefully cleaned *in situ* with live steam and/or chemical inactivation. Such cleaning media must not be exhausted into the atmosphere or be drained into ordinary sewers. After removal of such contaminated parts or equipment, they should be clearly tagged as to indicate the precautions needed in repair shops for subsequent manipulation.

Major problems will ensue when material sets hard in lines or equipment. After cleaning to the optimum degree possible, such equipment must be structurally isolated, e.g. by line *blanks,* for transport to specific areas designed to handle such contaminated fixtures. Here air supplied suits used in environmentally controlled enclosures should be used for final clean-up. However, where lines have become heavily loaded with hardened material their disposal is probably less expensive than the costs incurred in such difficult cleaning operations.

BIBLIOGRAPHY

Al'tganzen, *Cited by Temkin, I.S.*

Anon, Editorial: *Stilboestrol Cancer. Br Med J, 3*:593, 1971.

Amor, A.J.: *Growths of the Respiratory Tract* (Preliminary notice). Report of the VIII International Cong. for Industrial Accidents and Occupational Diseases. Leipz. 82:941, 1938 (Published 1939).

Arcos, J.C., Argus, M.F., and Wolf, G.: *Chemical Induction of Cancer.* New York, Academic Press, vol. I:431, 1968.

Askanazy, M.: Das experimentelle Karzinom. *Schweiz Med Wochenschr, 57*:1209, 1927.

Baetjer, A.M.: Pulmonary Carcinoma in Chromate Workers. *Arch Indust Hyg and Occup Med, 2*:505, 1950.

Barnes, J.M. and Magee, P.N.: Some toxic properties of dimethylnitrosamine. *Br J Ind Med, 11*:167, 1954.

Barnes, J.M., Benz, F.A., and Sisson, H.A.: Beryllium bone sarcomata in rabbits. *Br J Cancer, 4*:212, 1950.

Barsotti, M. and Vigliani, E.C.: Bladder lesions from aromatic amines: Statistical considerations and prevention. *Med Lav, 40*:129, 1949.

Baumslag, N., Keen, P., and Petering, H.G.: Carcinoma of the maxillary antrum and its relationship to trace metal content of snuff. *Arch Environ Health, 23*:1, 1971.

Battye, R.: Bladder carcinogens occurring during the production of "town" gas by coal carbonization. Proceedings of XV International Congress on Occupational Medicine. *3*:153, 1966.

Bidstrup, P.L. and Case, R.A.M.: Carcinoma of the lung in workmen in the biochromates producing industry in Great Britian. *Brit J Ind Med, 13*:260, 1956.

Billiard-Duschesne, J.L.: Amine induced tumours of the bladder. *J Urol Med Chir, 65*:784, 1959.

Bloom, A.D., Alva, A.A., Neriishi, S., Honda, T., and Archer, P.G.: Chromosome abberations in leukocytes of older survivors of the atomic bombings of Hiroshima and Nagasaki. *Lancet, 2*:802, 1967.

Bonser, G.M., Clayson, D.B., and Jull, J. Experimental enquiry into cause of industrial bladder cancer. *Lancet, 2*:286, 1951.

Bonser, G.M., Clayson, D.B., and Jull, J.W.: The induction of tumors of the subcutaneous tissues, liver and intestine in the mouse by certain dyestuffs and their intermediates. *Br J Cancer, 10*:653, 1956.

Bonser, G.M.: In Severi, L. (Ed.): *The Morphological Precursor of Cancer.* Perugia, 1962. p. 435.

89

Boyd, J.T., Doll, R., Faulds, J.S. and Leiper: Cancer of the lung in iron ore (hematite) miners. *Brit J Ind Med, 27*:97, 1970.

Braun, W.: Krebs an Haut und inneren Organen, Hervagerufen durch Arsen. *Dtsch Med Wochenschr, 83*:870, 1958.

Brinton, H.P., Frasier, E.S., and Koven, A.L.: Morbidity and mortality experience among chromate workers. *Public Health Repts, 67*:385, 1952.

Brock, N., Druckery, H., and Hamperl, H.: On the mode of action of carcinogenic chemicals. *Arch Exptl Pathol Pharmakol, 189*:709, 1938.

Brunsgaard, A.T.: Optreden av visse kreftformer blant gassverkarbeider. *Norske laegefor,* 755, 1959.

Bryan, W.R., and Shimkin, M.B.: Quantitative analysis of dose response data obtained with 3 carcinogenic hydrocarbons in 634 mice. *J National Cancer Inst, 3*:503, 1942-43.

Butt, L.T., and Stafford, N.: Papilloma of the bladder in the chemical industry. *J Appl Chem, 6*:525, 1956.

Cahan, W.G., Butler, F.S., Watson, W.L., and Pool, J.L.: Multiple cancers: Primary in the lung and other sites. *J Thorac Surg, 20*:335, 1950.

Campbell, J.A.: Effects of precipitated silica and of iron oxide on the incidence of primacy lung tumors in mice. *Br Med J, 2*:275, 1940.

Case, R.A.M., Hosker, M.E., McDonald, D.B., Pearson, H.T.: Tumors of the urinary bladder in workmen engaged in the manufacture and use of certain dyestuff intermediates in the British chemical industry, Part I. *Br J Ind Med, 11*:75, 1954.

Case, R.A.M. and Pearson, H.T.: Tumors of the urinary bladder in workmen engaged in the manufacture and use of certain dyestuff intermediates in the British chemical industry, Part II. *Br J Ind Med, 11*:213, 1954.

Cavigneaux, A., Delplace, Y., and Cabassin, G.: Les Statistiques de la Securite Sociale Concernant les affectures sanguines d'originne professionelle, 3 *eme* Journee de Pathol. Toxique, Paris, 1962.

Clayson, D.B.: Mode of carcinogenesis of armoatic amines. *Br J Cancer, 7*:460, 1953.

Clayson, D.B., Jull, J.W., and Bonser, G.M.: The testing of o-hydroxyamines and related compounds by bladder implantation and a discussion of their structural requirements for carcinogenicity. *Br J Cancer, 12*:222, 1958.

Clayson, D.B. and Ashton, M.: The metabolism of 1-naphthylamine and its bearing on the mode of carcinogenesis of the aromatic amines. *Acta Unio Contra Cancrum, 13*:539, 1963.

Clayson, D.B., Lawson, T.A., and Pringle, J.: The carcinogenic action of 2-aminodiphenylene oxide and 4-aminodiphenyl on the bladder and liver of the C57X IF mouse. *Br J Cancer, 21*:755, 1967.

Crabbe, J.G.S., Cresdee, W.C., Scott, T.S., and Williams, M.H.C.: The cytological diagnosis of bladder tumors amongst dyestuff workers. *Br J Ind Med, 13*:270, 1956.

Cramer, W., and Stowell, R.E.: On the quantitative evaluation of experimental carcinogenesis by methylcholanthrene. *Cancer Res, 3*:668, 1943.

Deichmann, W.B., Radomski, J.L., Anderson, W.S., Coplan, M.M., and Woods, F.M.: The carcinogenic action of p-aminobiphenyl in the dog. *Ind Med Surg, 27*:25, 1958a.

Deichmann, W.B., MacDonald, W.M., Coplan, M.M., Woods, R.M., and Anderson, W.A.D.: Paranitrobiphenyl, a new bladder carcinogen in the dog. *Ind Med Surg, 27*:634, 1958b.

Deichmann, W.B., Radomski, J.L., Glass, E., Anderson, W.A.D., Coplan, M.D., and Woods, F.M.: Synergism among oral carcinogens. Simultaneous feeding of four bladder carcinogens to dogs. *Ind Med Surg, 34*:640, 1965.

Den Engelise, L., Bentvelzen, P.A.J., and Emmelot, P.: Studies on lung tumors. I. *Chem-Biol. Interaction, 1*:395, 1970.

de Villiers, A.J., and Windish, J.P.: Lung cancer in a Fluospar mining community. *Br J Ind Med, 21*:94, 1964.

Doll, R.: Mortality from lung cancer among asbestos workers. *Br J Ind Med, 12*:81,1955.

Doll, R.: Cancer of the lung and nose in nickel workers. *Br J Ind Health 15*:217, 1958.

Doll, R., Fisher, R.E.W., Gammon, E.J., Gunn, W., Hughes, G.O., Tyrer, F.H., and Wilson, W.: Mortality of gas workers with special reference to cancers of the lung and bladder, chronic bronchitis and pneumoconcosis. *Br J Ind Med, 22*:1, 1965.

Druckerey, H., Schmähl, D., Dischler, W., and Schildback, A.: Dosis-Wirkungsbezichungen bei der Krebserzeugung durch 4-dimethylamine-stiben bei ratten. *Naturwizssenschftn, 49*:217, 1962.

Dunham, L.J. and Bailar, J.C.: World maps of cancer mortality rates and frequency ratios. *J Nat'l Cancer Inst, 41*:155, 1968.

Duggan, M.J., Soilleux, P.J., Strong, J.C. and Howell, D.M.: The exposure of United Kingdom miners to radon. *Br J Ind Med, 27*:106, 1970.

Dutra, F.R., Largent, E.J., and Roth, J.L.: Osteogenic sarcoma after inhalation of beryllium oxide. *AMA Arch Path, 51*:473, 1951.

Freund, H.A.: Clinical manifestations and studies in parenchymatous hepatitis. *Ann Intern Med, 10*:1144, 1937.

Girard, R., Tolot, F., and Bourrett, J.: Hydrocarbures benzeniques et hémopathies graves. *Arch Mal Prof, 31*:625, 1970.

Goguel, A., Cavingneaus, A., and Bernard, J.: Benzene induced leukemias in the Paris region between 1950 and 1965 (50 case observations). *Nouv Rev Fr Hematol, 7*:465, 1967.

Goldblatt, M.W.: Vesical tumours induced by chemical compounds. *Br J Ind Med, 6*:65, 1949.

Graham, J.B., Sotto, L.S.J. and Paloncek, F.P.: *Carcinoma of the cervix.* Philadephia, Saunders, 1967. pp. 94.

Greenwald, P., Barlow, J.J., Nasca, P.C., and Burnett, W.S.: Vaginal cancer after maternal treatment with synthetic estrogens. *N Eng J Med, 285*:390, 1971.

Gross, L., Gluckman, E.C., Kershaw, B.B., and Passelt, A.E.: Resistance of the white-foot field mouse to the carcinogenic action of urethane. *Cancer, 6*:124, 1953.

Gross, P., deTreville, R.T.P., Tolker, E., Kaschak, M., and Balyak, M.A.: Experimental asbestosis. *Arch Environ Health, 15*:343, 1967.

Grundmann, E., and Steinhoff, D.: Liver and lung tumors after 3,3'dichloro-4, 4'diaminodiphenylmethane in the rat. *Z Krebsforsch, 74*:28, 1970.

Haddow, A., and Horning, E.S.: On the carcinogenicity of an iron-dextran complex. *J Nat'l Cancer Inst, 24*:109, 1960.

Hendricks, N.V., Berry, C.M., Lione, J.G., and Thorpe, J.J.: Cancer of the scrotum in wax pressmen. I. Epidemiology. *Arch Environ Health, 19*:524, 1959.

Henry, S.A., and Irvine, E.D.: Cancer of the scrotum in the Blackburn registration district, 1837-1929. *J Hyg, 36*:310, 1936.

Henry, S.A.: The study of fatal cases of cancer of the scrotum from 1911 to 1935, with special reference to chimney sweeping and cotton mule spinning. *Am J Cancer, 3*:28, 1937.

Henry, S.A., Kennaway, E.L., and Kennaway, N.M.: The incidence of cancer of the bladder and prostate in certain occupations, *J Hyg* (Cambridge) *31*:125, 1931.

Hill, A.B., and Faning, E.C.: Studies in the incidence of cancer in a factory handling inorganic compounds of arsenic. I. mortality experience. *Br J Ind Med, 5*:2, 1948.

Horton, A.W., Denman, D.T., and Trosset, R.P.: Carcinogenesis of the skin. II. The accelerating properties of aliphatic and related hydrocarbons. *Cancer Res, 17*:758, 1957.

Hueper, W.C., Wiley, F.H., and Wolfe, H.D.: Experimental production of bladder tumours in dogs by administration of beta-naphthylamine. *J Indust Hyg Toxicol, 20*:45, 1938.

Hueper, W.C.: Experimental studies in cancerigenesis. *Arch Indust Health, 18*:284, 1958a.

Hueper, W.C.: Experimental studies in metal cancerigenesis. IX. *Arch Path,* (Chicago) *65*:600, 1958b.

Hueper, W.C., and Conway, W.D.: *Chemical Carcinogens and Cancers.* Springfield, Thomas, 1964.

Jones-Williams, W.: The pathology of the lungs in five nickel workers. *Br J Ind Med, 15*:235, 1958.

Kawai, M., Amamoto, H., and Harada, K.: Epidemiologic study of occupational lung cancer. *Arch Environ Health, 14*:859, 1967.

Kennaway, E.L., and Kennaway, N.M.: A further study of the incidence of cancer of the lung and larynx. *Br J Cancer, 1*:260, 1947.

Kopellmann, H., Robertson, M.H., Sanders, P.G., and Ash, I.: The Epping jaundice. *Br Med J, 1*:514, 1966.

Kopellmann, H., Scheuer, P.J., and Williams, R.: The liver lesion of the Epping jaundice. *Q J Med, 35*:553, 1966.

Kuroda, S., and Kawahata, K.: On the status of lung cancer among gas works employees. *Z Krebsfsch, 45*:36, 1936.

Laskin, S., Kuschner, M., and Drew, R.T.: Inhalation Carcinogenesis. AEC Symposium Ser. 18: U.S. Atomic Energy Commission, Washington, D.C., 1970.

Lee, A.M., and Fraumeni, J.F.: Arsenic and respiratory cancer in man. *J Nat'l Cancer Inst, 42*:1045, 1969.

Leitch, A., and Kennaway, E.L.: Experimental production of cancer by arsenic. *Br Med J, 2*:1107, 1922.

Lieben, J., and Williams, R.R.: Respiratory disease associated with beryllium refining and alloy fabrication. *J Occup Med, 11*:480, 1969.

Lignac, G.O.E.: Benzene leukemia in man and white mice. *Klin Wochenschr, 12*:109, 1933.

Lloyd, J.W.: Long term mortality study of steel workers, II, IV, V. *J Occup Med, 11*:299, 1969; *12*:151, 1970, *13*:53, 1971.

Løken, A.C.: Lungecarcinom hosnikkelarbeidere. *T norske Laegefor, 70*:376, 1950.

Machle, W., and Gregorius, F.: Cancer of the respiratory system in the U.S. chromate producing industry. *Public Health Repts, 63*:1114, 1948.

Magee, P.N., and Barnes, J.M.: The production of malignant primary hepatic tumors in the rat by feeding dimethylnitrosamine. *Br J Cancer, 10*:114, 1956.

Magee, P.N., and Barnes, J.M.: Induction of kidney tumors in the rat with dimethylnitrosamine. *J Pathol Bact, 84*:19, 1962.

Mancuso, T.F.: Occupational cancer and other health hazards in a chromate plant: A medical appraisal. II Clinical and toxicological approach. *Ind Med Surg, 20*:350, 393, 1951.

Mancuso, T.F., and El Attar, A.A.: A cohort study of workers exposed to beta-naphthylamine and benzidine. *J Occup Med, 9*:277, 1967.

Mancuso, T., and Coulter, F.J.: Methodology in industrial health studies. *Arch Environ Health, 6*:210, 1963.

Mancuso, T.F.: Relation of duration of employment and prior respiratory illness to respiratory cancer among beryllium workers. *Environ Res, 3*:251, 1970.

Mantel, N.: Symposium on chemical carcinogenesis. IV. The concept of threshhold in carcinogenesis. *Clin Pharmacol Ther, 4*:104, 1963.

Melamed, M.R., Koss, L.G., Ricci, A., and Whitmore, S.F.: Cytohistological observations on developing carcinoma of urinary bladder in man. *Cancer, 13*:67, 1960.

Melick, W.F., Escue, H.M., Naryka, J.J., Mezera, R.A., and Wheeler, E.R.: The first reported cases of human bladder tumors due to a new carcinogen - xenylamine *J Urol, 74*:760, 1955.

Melick, W.F., Naryka, J.J., and Kelly, R.E.: Bladder cancer due to exposure to p-aminobiphenyl: 17 year follow-up. *J Urol, 106*:220, 1971.

Merewether, E.R.A.: In Annual Rept. of the Chief Inspector of Factories for the Year 1947. H.M. Stationery Office, London, 1949.

Miller, J.A., and Miller, E.C.: The carcinogenic aminoazo dyes. *Adv Cancer Res, 1*:339, 1953.

Miller, J.A., and Miller, E.C.: Guest Editorial. Chemical carcinogenesis: Mechanisms—approaches to control. *J Nat'l Cancer Inst, 47*:V, 1971.

Moertel, C.G., Dockerty, M.B., and Baggenstoss, A.J.: Multiple primary malignant neoplasms. III. Tumors of multicentric origin. *Cancer, 14*:238, 1961.

Monlibert, L., and Roubile, R.: A propos der cancer bronchique chez le mineur de fer. *J Franc Med Chur Thor, 14*:435, 1960.

Monnier-Williams, G.S.: *Trace Elements in Food.* London, Butler and Taylor, Ltd., 1949.

Morgan, J.G.: Some observations on the incidence of respiratory cancer in nickel workers. *Br J Ind Med, 15*:224, 1958.

Morris, H.G., Dubnik, C.S., and Johnson, J.M.: Studies in carcinogenic studies in rat of 2 nitro-, 2 amino-, 2 acetylamino-and 2 deacetylamino fluorene after ingestion and after painting. *J Nat'l Cancer Inst, 10*:1201, 1950.

Müller, A.: Uber Blasenveränderungen durch Amine. *Z Urol Chirg, 36*:202, 1933.

Müller, A.: Uber Blasen-und Nierenschädigungen der Farbstoffindustrie. *Helv Chir Acta, 18*:1, 1951.

Munn, A.: *Bladder Cancer.* K.F. Lampe, Ed., Birmingham, Aesculapius, 1967, p. 187.

Napolkov, N.P., and Alexandrov, V.A.: On the effects of blastomogenic substances on the organism during embryogenesis. *Ztschrf f Krebsforsch, 71*:32, 1968.

Osburn, H.S.: Cancer of the lung in Gwanda. *Cent Afr J Med, 3*:215, 1957.

Passay, R.D.: Experimental soot cancer. *Br Med J, 2*:1112, 1922.

Pfieffer, A.O., and Allen, E.: Attempts to produce cancer in Rhesus monkeys with carcinogenic hydrocarbons and estrogens. *Cancer Res 8*:97, 1948.

Pinto, S.S., and Bennett, B.M.: Effect of arsenic trioxide exposure on mortality. *Arch Environ Health, 7*:583, 1963.

Pliss, G.B.: Concerning carcinogenous properties of o-tolidine and dianisidine. *Gig Tr Prof Zabol, 9*:18, 1965.

Pliss, G.B.: Experimental tumors induced in rats by dichlorobenzidine. *Vaprosy Oncol, 5*:524, 1959.

Pliss, G.B., and Zabezhinsby, M.A.: Carcinogenic properties of o-tolidine. *J Nat'l Cancer Inst, 45*:283, 1970.

Poole-Wilson, D.S.: In Riches, E.W. (Ed.): *Modern Trends in Urology.* London, Butterworth, 1953.

Report of the Advisory Committee to the Surgeon General of the Public Health Service: Smoking and Health, PHS. Publication. No. 1103, U.S. Dept of Health, Education and Welfare, 1964.

Roth, F.: Uber den Bronchialkrebs arsengeschadigter winzer. *Virchow's Arch Pathol Anat, 331*:119, 1958.

Roussel, J., Pernot, C., Schoumacher, P., Pernot, M., and Kesslee, Y.: Statistical considerations regarding bronchiogenic cancer among iron miners in the Lorraine basin. *J Radiol Electrol Med Nucl, 45*:541, 1965.

Saffotti, U.F., Kolb, L.H., and Shubik, P.: Experimental studies of the conditions of exposure to carcinogenics for lung cancer induction. *J Am Pollut Control Assoc, 15*:23, 1965.

Schepers, G.W.H., Durkan, T.M., Delehant, A.B., and Creedon, F.T.: The biological action of inhaled beryllium sulfate. *Arch Ind Health, 15*:23, 1957.

Schmorl, G.: Pathological study of Schneeberg lung cancer. *Rept Int'l Conf on Cancer,* London, 1928. John Wright and Sons, Ltd., Bristol, 1928, p. 272.

Schoental, R.: Carcinogenic and chronic effects of 4,4'diaminodiphenyl methane, an expoxyresin. *Nature* (London), *219*:1162, 1968.

Schoenthal, R.: Pathological lesions, including tumors, in rats after 4, 4'diaminodiphenyl methane and gamma butyrolactone. *Is J Med Sci, 4*:1146, 1968.

Sciarini, L.J., and Meigs, J.W.: Biotransformation of the benzidines, III. *Arch Environ Health, 2*:584, 1961.

Scott, T.S., and Williams, MHC.: The control of industrial bladder tumours. *Br J Ind Med, 14*:150, 1957.

Scott, T.S.: *Carcinogenic and Chronic Toxic Hazards of Aromatic Amines.* Amsterdam, *Elsevier,* 1962, p. 208.

Selikoff, I.J., Churg, J., and Hammond, E.C.: The occurrance of asbestosis among insulation workers in the United States. *Ann NY Acad Sci, 132*:139, 1965.

Sellakumar, A.R., Montesano, R., and Saffiotti, V.: Aromatic amines carcinogenicity in hamsters. *Proc Amer Assoc Cancer Res, 10*:78, 1969.

Shubik, P.: *Biological determination of the action of chemical carcinogens.* In Proc. 4th Nat'l. Cancer Conf. Minneapolis, Sept. 13-15, 1960. Lippincott, p. 113.

Smith, W.E., Sunderland, D.A., and Sugma, K.: Experimental analysis of the carcinogenic activity of certain petroleum products. *AMA Arch Ind Hyg Occup Med, 4*:299, 1951.

Snegreff, L.S., and Lombard, O.M.: Arsenic and cancer. *Arch Ind Hyg, 4*:199, 1951.

Spitz, S., Maguigan, W.H., and Dobriner, K.: The carcinogenic action of benzidine. *Cancer, 3*:789, 1950.

Stagg, H.E., and Reed, R.H.: The determination of 4-aminodiphenyl in technical diphenylamine. *Analyst, 82*:503, 1957.

Strait, L.A., Horenoff, M.K., and DeOme, K.B.: The influence of solvents upon the effectiveness of carcinogenic agents. *Cancer Res 8*:231, 1948.

Sunderman, F.W., Donnely, A.J., and West, B.: Nickel poisoning. IV. Chronic exposure to rats to nickel carbonyl. *Arch Ind Health, 16*:480, 1957.

Sutherland, R.B. (1959) cf. Doll, R.: Occupational lung cancer: A review. *Br J Ind Med, 16*:181, 1959.

Syverton, J.T., Berry, J.P., and Dascomb, H.E.: Studies on carcinogenesis in rabbits. *Cancer Res, 2*:436, 1942.

Tannenbaum, A.: Contribution of urethane studies to the understanding of carcinogenesis. In National Cancer Inst. Monograph No. 14, 341, U.S. Dept. of Health, Education and Welfare, Bethesda, Maryland, May, 1964.

Temken, I.S.: *Industrial Bladder Carcinogenesis* (English Translation) Pergamon Press, Oxford, 1963, p. 33.

Tepper, L.B., Hardy, H.L., and Chamberlin, R.L.: Toxicity of Beryllium Compounds. Amsterdam, Elsevier, 1961.

Terracini, B., Shubik, P., and Della Porta, G.: A study of skin carcinogenesis in the mouse with single applications of 9,10 dimethy-1,2-benzanthracene at different dosages. *Cancer Res, 20*:1538, 1966.

Troll, W., and Nelson, N.: Studies on aromatic amines. I Preliminary observations on benzidine metabolism. *Am Ind Hyg Assoc J, 19*:499, 1958.

Twort, C.C., and Twort, J.M.: The carcinogenic potency of mineral oils. *J Ind Hyg, 13*:204, 1931.

Vigliani, E.C., and Saita, G.: Benzene and leukemia. *New Engl J Med, 271*:872, 1964.

Vorwald, A.J., Reeves, A.L., and Urban, E.C.J.: In, *Beryllium—Its Industrial Hygiene Aspects,* Academic Press 1966, p. 201.

Wada, S., Miyanishi, M., Nichimoto, K., Kambe, S., and Miller, R.N.: Mustard gas as a cause of respiratory neoplasia in man. *Lancet, 1*:1161, 1968.

Wagner, J.C.: The sequellae of exposure to asbestos dust. *Ann NY Acad Sci, 132*:691, 1965.

Walpole, A.L.: On substances inducing cancer of the bladder. *Acta Unio contra cancrum, 19*:483, 1963.

Walpole, A.L., Williams, M.H.C., and Roberts, D.C.: Tumors of the urinary bladder of dogs after ingestion of 4-aminodiphenyl. *Br J Ind Med, 11*:105, 1954.

Washburn, V.: The treatment of aniline tumours of the urinary bladder. *J Urol, 38*:232, 1937.

Weil, C.S., Carpenter, C.P., and Symth, H.J., Jr.: Urinary bladder response to diethylene glycol. *Arch Environ Health, 11*:569, 1965.

Weil-Malherbe, H., and Dickens, F.: Factors affecting carcinogenesis IV. The effect of tricaprylin solutions of cholesterol and phospholiins. *Cancer Res, 6*:171, 1946.

WHO, Manual of the International Statistical Classification of Disease, Injuries and Causes of Death, (WHO), Geneva, Seventh Revision, 1957.

WHO Statistics Report 23:126, 1970.

Williams, M.H.C., and Bonser, G.M.: Induction of hepatomas in rats and mice following the administration of auramine. *Br J Cancer, 16*:87, 1962.

Wolfe, H.D.: Routine cystoscopic examination as a control measure in anilin tumor of the bladder. *J Urol, 38*:216, 1937.

Wynder, E.L., Spranger, J.W., and Fark, M.M.: Dose-response studies with benzo (a)pyrene. *Cancer, 13*:106, 1960.

INDEX